LEAN AND GREEN AIR FRYER COOKBOOK

120 AFFORDABLE, QUICK & EASY AIR FRYER RECIPES. 30-DAY MEAL PLAN INCLUDED. | 1000 DAYS FUELING HACKS TO HELP YOU KEEP HEALTHY AND LOSE WEIGHT.

PAMELA KENDRICK

CONTENTS

Introduction ix
Optavia Diet Basics xi

BREAKFAST

1. Cheesy Egg Bites — 3
2. Egg & Pepper — 5
3. Spinach Egg Muffins — 7
4. Parmesan Spinach Egg Muffins — 9
5. Cheddar Kale Egg Cups — 11
6. Mushroom Spinach Egg Muffins — 13
7. Easy Scrambled Eggs — 15
8. Egg & Tomato — 17
9. Healthy Spinach Frittata — 19
10. Vegetable Egg Muffins — 21

LEAN & GREEN POULTRY

11. Delicious No Breading Chicken Breast — 25
12. Lemon Pepper Chicken Breast — 27
13. Flavorful Chicken Fajita — 29
14. Juicy & Crispy Chicken Wings — 31
15. Spice Herb Chicken Breast — 33
16. Spicy Meatballs — 35
17. Herb Garlic Butter Chicken Wings — 37
18. Flavorful Chicken Drumsticks — 39
19. Tasty Chicken Thighs — 41
20. Orange Honey Chicken Wings — 43
21. Garlic Butter Turkey Breast — 45
22. Meatballs — 47
23. Dry Rub Chicken Drumsticks — 49

24. Juicy Lemon Chicken Thighs	51
25. Easy & Super Moist Chicken Wings	53
26. Rosemary Turkey Breast	55
27. Tender Turkey Legs	57
28. Meatballs	59
29. Delicious Chicken Patties	61
30. Herb Turkey Breast	63
31. BBQ Chicken Breast	65
32. Chicken Fritters	66
33. Greek Chicken	68
34. Easy Lemon Chicken	70
35. Meatballs	71
36. Garlic Herb Chicken Breast	73
37. Meatballs	75
38. Coconut Turkey Meatballs	77
39. Cheesy Chicken Meatballs	79
40. Meatballs	81

LEAN & GREEN PORK

41. Easy Pork Patties	85
42. Lemon Pepper Pork Chops	87
43. Meatballs	88
44. Crispy Crusted Parmesan Pork Chops	90
45. Spicy Pork Steak	92
46. Dash Pork Chops	94
47. Juicy Pork Chops	95
48. Creole Pork Chops	97
49. Cajun Pork Chops	99
50. Flavorful Lemon Garlic Pork Chops	101
51. Thyme Garlic Pork Chops	103
52. Pesto Pork Chops	105
53. Spicy Garlic Pork Chops	106
54. Meatballs	108
55. Flavorful Spicy Pork Chops	110

LEAN & GREEN SEAFOOD

56. Flavorful Prawns	115
57. Lemon Garlic Shrimp	117
58. Old Bay Spicy Shrimp	119
59. Lemon Garlic Salmon	121
60. Parmesan Herb Crust Salmon	123
61. Simple Paprika Salmon	125
62. Crab Patties	127
63. Air Fried Catfish Fillets	129
64. Simple Lime Garlic Shrimp	131
65. Crispy Coconut Shrimp	133
66. Basil Parmesan Shrimp	135
67. Parmesan Cajun Shrimp	137
68. Sriracha Shrimp	139
69. Chili Garlic Shrimp	141
70. Quick Salmon Patties	143
71. Delicious Asian Shrimp	145
72. Garlic Rosemary Shrimp	147
73. Greek Shrimp	149
74. Simple Cajun Shrimp	151
75. Spicy Lemon Shrimp	153
76. Lemon Pepper Tilapia	155
77. Herb Tuna Patties	157
78. Simple Cajun Salmon	159
79. Quick Salmon Burger Patties	160
80. Herb Fish Fillets	162
81. Marinated Asian Salmon	164
82. Old Bay Salmon	166
83. Lemon Pepper White Fish	168
84. Delicious Herb Salmon	170
85. Flavorful Spicy Shrimp	172
86. Simple Shrimp Fajitas	174
87. Lemon Pepper Basa	176
88. Spicy Halibut	178
89. Air Fry Catfish Fillets	180
90. Lemon Garlic Swordfish	182
91. Simple Garlic Tilapia	184
92. Spicy Cod	186
93. Garlic Rosemary Shrimp	188
94. Flavors Parmesan Shrimp	190
95. Shrimp with Vegetables	192

GREEN & SIDE DISHES

96. Healthy & Tasty Green Beans	197
97. Cheesy Brussels Sprouts	199
98. Garlic Cauliflower Florets	201
99. Delicious Ratatouille	203
100. Simple Green Beans	205
101. Air Fryer Tofu	207
102. Healthy Zucchini Patties	209
103. Healthy Asparagus Spears	211
104. Spicy Brussels Sprouts	213
105. Cheese Broccoli Fritters	215
106. Air Fryer Bell Peppers	217
107. Air Fried Tasty Eggplant	219
108. Asian Green Beans	221
109. Spicy Asian Brussels Sprouts	222
110. Healthy Mushrooms	224
111. Cheese Stuff Peppers	226
112. Cheesy Broccoli Cauliflower	228
113. Air Fryer Broccoli & Brussels Sprouts	230
114. Spicy Asparagus Spears	232
115. Stuffed Mushrooms	234
116. Broccoli Tots	236
117. Cheesy Jalapeno Pepper	238
118. Tasty Eggplant Slices	240
119. Healthy Zucchini Chips	242
120. Rosemary Basil Mushrooms	244
30-Day Meal Plan	246
Conclusion	251

© **Copyright 2021 by Pamela Kendrick. All Rights Reserved.**

In no way is it legal to reproduce, duplicate, or transmit any part of this document by either electronic means or in printed format. Recording of this publication is strictly prohibited, and any storage of this material is not allowed unless with written permission from the publisher. All rights reserved.

The information provided herein is stated to be truthful and consistent, in that any liability, regarding inattention or otherwise, by any usage or abuse of any policies, processes, or directions contained within is the solitary and complete responsibility of the recipient reader. Under no circumstances will any legal liability or blame be held against the publisher for any reparation, damages, or monetary loss due to the information herein, either directly or indirectly.

Respective authors own all copyrights not held by the publisher.

Legal Notice:

This book is copyright protected. This is only for personal use. You cannot amend, distribute, sell, use, quote or paraphrase any part of the content within this book without the consent of the author or copyright owner. Legal action will be pursued if this is breached.

Disclaimer Notice:

Please note the information contained within this document is for educational and entertainment purposes only. Every attempt has been made to provide accurate, up-to-date and reliable, complete information. No warranties of any kind are expressed or implied. Readers acknowledge that the author is not engaging in the rendering of legal, financial, medical or professional advice.

By reading this document, the reader agrees that under no circumstances are we responsible for any losses, direct or indirect, which are incurred as a result of the use of information contained within this document, including, but not limited to, errors, omissions, or inaccuracies.

INTRODUCTION

The Optavia diet is driven and introduces by Medifast, is a famous food substitute company. The Optavia diet program requires feed you low carb and low-calorie food. The Optavia diet is one of the effective weight loss which reduces your weight rapidly and offers you long term weight loss benefits. To lose your weight effectively you have to consume packaged food provided by the company with a homemade green bean meal. The packaged food or mini-meals provided by the company is also known as fuelings.

    The fuelings are made up of more than 60 items which are low in carb and high in proteins and probiotics culture. Probiotics are one kind of good bacteria that helps to boost your gut health and also improves your digestive system. The Optavia diet is one of the best choices for busy lifestyle people who want to lose their weight but don't have time to cook your meal. The Optavia diet not only loses your weight but also helps to change your eating habits towards healthy eating. The company not only supplies you with healthy foods but also provide you trainers and useful information regarding diet plans. To get fast weight loss benefits the trainer recommends doing at least 30 minutes of exercise daily.

Introduction

The Optavia diet is one of the most preferred diets in the United States. If you want to adopt the Optavia diet and want to enjoy the benefits of the diet then this book will guide you about the diet and also loaded with healthy and delicious Optavia diet recipes.

The cookbook contains Optavia recipes written from different categories like breakfast, lean and green poultry, lean and green pork, lean and green seafood, and green & side. All the recipes written in this book are unique and written into easily understandable form with step by step instructions. It also comes with preparation and cooking time. All the recipes end with their nutritional value information. The nutritional value information is used to calculate your daily carb and calorie consumption during the Optavia diet. There is various type of cookbooks available in the market on this topic thanks of choosing my book. I hope you love and enjoy all the recipes written in this cookbook.

OPTAVIA DIET BASICS

What is the Optavia Diet?
　The Optavia diet is one of the effective weight loss diet followed by many people to reduce their excess body weight. The Optavia is a meal replacement plan in which you have to consume low calorie and reduced carb packaged foods with one homemade lean and green meal. The Optavia diet program driven by a Medifast, which is one of the meal replacement company. The Optavia diet is fundamentally a version of the Medifast diet plan. In this plan, dieters eat a certain amount of mini-meals provided by the company is called fuelings.
　The Optavia fueling contains more than 60 food items which are low in calories and high in proteins. It also contains probiotics which are one kind of microorganism having many health benefits. You may also call it friendly bacteria which help to improve your gut health. These fueling food items include bars, shakes, cookies, soups, puddings, pasta, cereals, and more. Optavia diet is not a cheap diet plan but most health-conscious people prefer to follow this diet for effective and fast weight loss purposes. You can easily lose your body weight by consuming low-calorie food throughout the day.

Optavia Diet Basics

The Optavia diet is not only using to reduce weight but also changes your unhealthy eating habits towards healthy eating. The Optavia diet is also very beneficial for those people who suffer from type-2 diabetes, gouts, and senior citizens people. Most of the research and studies published in journals show that the people follow the Optavia diet plan notice the significant health benefits within 8 weeks.

Optavia Diet Programs

The Optavia diet offers three types of different diet programs. Among these three diet programs, you can choose any program according to your health needs. The first two programs are used for weight loss purposes and the third program is used for weight maintenance.

Optimal weight 5&1 Plan

Most of the people follows the optimal weight 5&1 plan for weight loss purpose. Following this diet plan, you can drop down near about 12 pounds weight within 12 weeks. This plan offers you to eat 5 Optavia fuelings with one lean and green meal every day.

Optimal weight 4&2&1 Plan

This plan is one of the best choices for those peoples who want more flexibility or calories in their food choices. The plan offers four Optavia fuelings, two lean and green meals, and one healthy snack each day. It allows eating six times daily within two to three hours of gap.

Optimal weight 3&3 Plan

This plan offers nutritionally balanced small meals designed for maintenance purposes. The plan offers three Optavia fueling and three lean and green meals. It is recommended that to eat a small portion of meals every two to three hours of the day.

The Optavia Company offers additional tools such as mobile apps which helps to keep track of your daily food intake and activities. You can also set the meal reminders with the help of an app. Apart from this company sends inspirational text messages, gives tips via community forums, and more to support weight loss and weight maintenance.

What to Eat on Optavia Diet?

The daily food consumption is depending upon which type of diet plan you have chosen. Most of these pre-packaged foods come from the company in the form of fuelings. You have to eat a daily meal as per the given number of lean and green meals which consist of non-starchy veggies and lean protein. The types of food list which allows during Optavia diet are given as follows:

Optavia Fueling

The Optavia fueling is made up of high-quality protein which helps to maintain lean muscle mass. It also comes with probiotics, which is one kind of good bacteria that helps to improve your digestive health. Optavia fueling consists of 60 nutritious, healthy, and delicious fuelings include bars, soups, cookies, puddings, shakes, brownies, pretzels, and more. You can consume all these fuels alternatively as per your diet plan suggest.

Lean Meats

Lean meats are low-fat meat. The lean and green meal contains 5 to 7 ounces of lean protein with non-starchy vegetables. The Optavia diet divides lean meat into three different categories

1. **Lean Meat:** Lean meat includes pork chops, salmon and lamb
2. **Leaner Meat:** Leaner Meat categories include sward fish and chicken breast.
3. **Leanest Meat:** Shrimps and cod are comes under these categories.

Non-Starchy and green vegetables

The non-starchy vegetables again divided into three different categories

Low carb veggies: This category includes green salads.

1. Moderate carb veggies: Summer squash and cauliflower are comes under this category.
2. High carb veggies: Peppers and broccoli come under

the high carb category.

Healthy fats

It is recommended to use healthy fats during the Optavia diet. These healthy fats include polyunsaturated and monounsaturated fats which are healthier fats than saturated fats olive oil, flaxseed oil, walnut oil, avocado oil are some examples of healthy fats allowed during the Optavia diet. You have to consume 0 to 2 servings of healthy fats with a lean green meal from these categories.

Weight Maintenance

When you are achieving your weightless goal then you have to shift 3&3 plan to maintain your healthy body weight. You can consume fresh fruits, low-fat dairy products, meatless alternatives, and whole grain to maintain an ideal weight.

Tips to Follow the Optavia Diet

The Optavia diet gives weight loss benefits to their dieters. The success of any diet depends on how you follow the diet regimen. To follow the Optavia diet successfully just follows the tips given below.

- Always cook your food with a healthy cooking method like broiling, grilling, baking, poaching, and air frying method. Avoid unhealthy deep frying methods of cooking which raise your calories.
- Consume portion size recommended as per diet plan. The actual portion size is measured when it is cooked.
- Select the foods that are rich in Omega-3 fatty acids which help to lower the inflammation. It also helps to improve your heart health. These foods include salmon, trout, mackerel, herring, and other fishes especially cold water fishes.
- If you find the alternatives for meat then choose the tofu or tempeh. These foods are low in calories and high in protein.
- Strictly follow the program for its success. If you are

Optavia Diet Basics

dining out then also prefer a healthy and nutritious meal. During the diet period keep away from alcohol consumption, it may be kicking out you from the diet.

The Benefits of Optavia Diet

The Optavia diet is one of the effective weight-loss diets. The U.S News & World Report ranked the Optavia diet at second position for its fastest weight loss categories. There are various benefits of following the diet. These benefits are given as follows:

Effective Weight loss

When you follow the Optavia 5&1 diet plan your carb and calorie intake is reduced and it also helps to control the portion size of the meal. It also limits your daily calorie consumption in the range of 800 to 1000 calories each day and divides these calories from six meal portions. The obesity science and practice conducted a 16-week study over 198 people who following the Optavia 5&1 diet plan. During the study, they have noticed significant weight loss, reduction in the fat level, and reduce waist circumference compared with other diet groups.

It is easy to follow

As compare to other diets Optavia diet is less restrictive and easy to follow. The Optavia diet offers a structured eating plan and all the information given on their site will help you to easily follow the diet. The diet mostly depends on company packaged fuelings. If you follow the 5&1 plan then you have to cook only one meal per day. A simple meal plan makes Optavia diet easy to follow. If you don't have time to cook your lean and green meals at home then you can buy packaged meals known as the flavor of home.

Helps to improve Blood pressure

When you are on the Optavia diet your sodium intake is limited and due to weight loss it helps to improve your blood pressure level. The 40-week study conducted over 90 peoples who are facing the obesity issue shows rapid weight reduction and blood pressure level.

It offers long-term ongoing supports

This is one of the great things while you are following the Optavia diet. The diet coaches are available to guide you throughout the year. The coaches help you by delivering proper guidance and inspire you to achieve your weight loss goal and also help in body maintenance during the diet period.

FAQs
Is exercise necessary during the Optavia diet?

Exercise is one of the necessary parts when you want to lose weight. It helps to improve your metabolic process to maintain weight loss. To get better results you must exercise during the diet.

Which is the best program for me?

The Optavia diet has different types of programs designed for a different purpose. Some are used for weight loss purposes and some for weight maintenance purposes. It depends on your need and your health conditions. The better way to talk with your Optavia coach.

Should I take a multivitamin supplement during the diet?

No need to take any multi-vitamin supplement during the diet because the Optavia diet includes more than 24 vitamins and minerals which is essential to keep you fit and healthy.

What is a lean and green meal in diet?

The meal which contains 5 to 7 ounce of cooked lean protein with 3 servings of non-starchy green vegetables and 2 servings of healthy fat is known as a lean and green meal.

What exactly fueling means?

Fueling is one kind of mini-meal provided by the Optavia diet company. The fueling contains high-quality lean protein and friendly bacteria which helps to improve your gut health. Fueling food includes bars, shakes, soups, biscuits, puddings, and more.

Can I consume alcohol during the diet?

No, because alcohol is responsible to increase carb and calorie intake. This will kick out you from the fat burning process and weight loss process. It also responsible for dehydration, increase calories, decrease inhabitation, and doesn't contain any nutritional value. Strictly avoid alcohol during the diet.

BREAKFAST

1

CHEESY EGG BITES

Preparation Time: 10 minutes
Cooking Time: 5 minutes
Serve: 4

Ingredients:
- 4 eggs
- ¼ cup cheddar cheese, shredded
- ¼ tsp garlic powder
- ¼ cup heavy cream
- Pepper
- Salt

Directions:
1. In a bowl, whisk eggs with garlic powder, cheese, heavy cream, pepper, and salt.
2. Pour egg mixture into the four silicone muffin molds.
3. Place molds in the air fryer basket and cook at 350 F for 5 minutes.
4. Serve and enjoy.

Nutritional Value (Amount per Serving):
- Calories 117

- Fat 9.5 g
- Carbohydrates 0.7 g
- Sugar 0.4 g
- Protein 7.5 g
- Cholesterol 181 mg

2
EGG & PEPPER

Preparation Time: 10 minutes
Cooking Time: 5 minutes
Serve: 4

Ingredients:
- 4 eggs
- 2 bell peppers, cut in half & remove seeds
- 4 bacon slices, cooked & crumbled
- ½ cup cheddar cheese, shredded
- Pepper
- Salt

Directions:
1. In a bowl, whisk eggs with pepper and salt. Stir in cheese and bacon.
2. Pour egg mixture into the four bell pepper halves.
3. Place bell pepper halves in the air fryer basket and cook at 350 F for 5 minutes.
4. Serve and enjoy.

Nutritional Value (Amount per Serving):
- Calories 143

PAMELA KENDRICK

- Fat 9.6 g
- Carbohydrates 5.1 g
- Sugar 3.4 g
- Protein 9.8 g
- Cholesterol 179 mg

3

SPINACH EGG MUFFINS

Preparation Time: 10 minutes
Cooking Time: 15 minutes
Serve: 6

Ingredients:
- 3 eggs
- 1 cup fresh spinach, chopped
- 3 bacon slices, cooked & crumbled
- ½ cup cheddar cheese, shredded
- ¼ tsp baking powder
- 2 tbsp heavy cream
- ¼ tsp pepper
- ¼ tsp salt

Directions:
1. In a bowl, whisk eggs with heavy cream, pepper, baking powder, and salt.
2. Stir in spinach, bacon, and cheese.
3. Pour egg mixture into the 6 silicone muffin molds.
4. Place muffin molds into the air fryer basket and cook at 350 F for 15-18 minutes or until eggs are set.
5. Serve and enjoy.

Nutritional Value (Amount per Serving):
- Calories 140
- Fat 11.2 g
- Carbohydrates 0.9 g
- Sugar 0.3 g
- Protein 8.9 g
- Cholesterol 109 mg

4

PARMESAN SPINACH EGG MUFFINS

Preparation Time: 10 minutes
Cooking Time: 15 minutes
Serve: 6

Ingredients:
- 6 eggs
- ½ tsp red pepper flakes
- 2 tbsp parmesan cheese, shredded
- 2.5 oz baby spinach, chopped
- Pepper
- Salt

Directions:
1. In a bowl, whisk eggs with red pepper flakes, pepper, and salt.
2. Stir in parmesan cheese and spinach.
3. Pour egg mixture into the 6 silicone muffin molds.
4. Place muffin molds into the air fryer basket and cook at 325 F for 15 minutes or until eggs are set.
5. Serve and enjoy.

Nutritional Value (Amount per Serving):
- Calories 70

- Fat 4.7 g
- Carbohydrates 0.9 g
- Sugar 0.4 g
- Protein 6.2 g
- Cholesterol 164 mg

5

CHEDDAR KALE EGG CUPS

Preparation Time: 10 minutes
Cooking Time: 15 minutes
Serve: 6

Ingredients:
- 5 eggs
- 3 oz cheddar cheese, shredded
- 1 cup kale, chopped
- Pepper
- Salt

Directions:
1. In a bowl, whisk eggs with pepper and salt.
2. Stir in cheese and kale.
3. Pour egg mixture into the 6 silicone muffin molds.
4. Place muffin molds into the air fryer basket and cook at 325 F for 15 minutes or until eggs are set.
5. Serve and enjoy.

Nutritional Value (Amount per Serving):
- Calories 115
- Fat 8.3 g

- Carbohydrates 1.6 g
- Sugar 0.4 g
- Protein 8.5 g
- Cholesterol 151 mg

6

MUSHROOM SPINACH EGG MUFFINS

Preparation Time: 10 minutes
Cooking Time: 5 minutes
Serve: 6

Ingredients:
- 6 egg
- 1 cup Asiago cheese, shredded
- 2 tbsp milk
- ½ tbsp olive oil
- ½ cup spinach, chopped
- 3 oz mushrooms, sliced
- Pepper
- Salt

Directions:
1. Heat oil in a pan over medium heat.
2. Add mushroom to the pan and sauté until softened. Add spinach and cook until spinach is wilted.
3. Divide spinach mushroom mixture into the 6 silicone muffin molds.
4. In a bowl, whisk eggs with milk, pepper, and salt. Stir in cheese.

5. Pour egg mixture over vegetables into each muffin mold.

6. Place muffin molds into the air fryer basket and cook at 325 F for 15-18 minutes or until eggs are set.

7. Serve and enjoy.

Nutritional Value (Amount per Serving):
- Calories 159
- Fat 12.4 g
- Carbohydrates 2.5 g
- Sugar 0.8 g
- Protein 11.6 g
- Cholesterol 184 mg

7

EASY SCRAMBLED EGGS

Preparation Time: 10 minutes
Cooking Time: 6 minutes
Serve: 2

Ingredients:
- 4 eggs
- 1 tbsp parmesan cheese, grated
- 1/2 tsp garlic powder
- Pepper
- Salt

Directions:
1. Whisk eggs with garlic powder, pepper, and salt. Stir in cheese.
2. Pour egg mixture into the air fryer baking dish.
3. Place dish in the air fryer and cook at 360 F for 2 minutes.
4. Remove baking dish from air fryer and stir quickly and air fry for 4 minutes more.
5. Stir and serve.

Nutritional Value (Amount per Serving):
- Calories 150

- Fat 9.1 g
- Carbohydrates 4.5 g
- Sugar 1.1 g
- Protein 11 g
- Cholesterol 325 mg

8
EGG & TOMATO

Preparation Time: 10 minutes
Cooking Time: 25 minutes
Serve: 2

Ingredients:
- 2 eggs
- 2 large tomatoes, cut top & scoop out innards
- 1/4 tsp garlic powder
- Pepper
- Salt

Directions:
1. Preheat the air fryer to 325 F.
2. In a bowl, whisk eggs with garlic powder, pepper, and salt.
3. Pour egg mixture into each tomato.
4. Place tomato in the air fryer basket and cook for 25 minutes.
5. Serve and enjoy.

Nutritional Value (Amount per Serving):
- Calories 96
- Fat 5 g
- Carbohydrates 7.5 g

PAMELA KENDRICK

- Sugar 5 g
- Protein 7 g
- Cholesterol 164 mg

9

HEALTHY SPINACH FRITTATA

Preparation Time: 10 minutes
Cooking Time: 8 minutes
Serve: 1

Ingredients:
- 3 eggs
- 1 cup spinach, chopped
- 2 tbsp cheddar cheese, grated
- 1 small onion, minced
- Pepper
- Salt

Directions:
1. Preheat the air fryer to 350 F.
2. In a bowl, whisk eggs with the remaining ingredients.
3. Pour egg mixture into the greased air fryer pan.
4. Place pan in the air fryer basket and cook for 8 minutes or until eggs are set.
5. Serve and enjoy.

Nutritional Value (Amount per Serving):
- Calories 385

- Fat 23.3 g
- Carbohydrates 10.7 g
- Sugar 4.1 g
- Protein 34.3 g
- Cholesterol 520 mg

10

VEGETABLE EGG MUFFINS

Preparation Time: 10 minutes
Cooking Time: 20 minutes
Serve: 4

Ingredients:
- 4 eggs
- 4 tbsp half and half
- 1 cup mixed vegetables, diced
- 1 cup cheddar cheese, shredded
- Pepper
- Salt

Directions:
1. In a bowl, whisk eggs with half and half, 1/2 cup cheese, pepper, and salt. Stir in vegetables.
2. Pour egg mixture into the four silicone muffin molds.
3. Place muffin molds in the air fryer basket and cook at 300 F for 12 minutes.
4. Top with remaining cheese and cook at 400 F for 2 minutes.
5. Serve and enjoy.

Nutritional Value (Amount per Serving):
- Calories 195

- Fat 11 g
- Carbohydrates 6 g
- Sugar 0.5 g
- Protein 13 g
- Cholesterol 190 mg

LEAN & GREEN POULTRY

11

DELICIOUS NO BREADING CHICKEN BREAST

Preparation Time: 10 minutes
Cooking Time: 14 minutes
Serve: 6

Ingredients:
- 1 ½ lbs chicken breasts, skinless and boneless
- For marinade:
- ¼ tsp cayenne
- ½ tsp pepper
- 1 tsp Italian seasoning
- 1 tsp coconut aminos
- 1 tbsp fresh lemon juice
- 1 tbsp Dijon mustard
- ½ cup mayonnaise
- 1 tsp sea salt

Directions:
1. Add chicken into the large zip-lock bag. Mix all marinade ingredients and pour over chicken in a zip-lock bag. Seal bag and place in the refrigerator for 1 hour.
2. Preheat the air fryer to 400.

3. Place marinated chicken breasts into the air fryer basket and cook for 14 minutes. Turn chicken halfway through.

4. Serve and enjoy.

Nutritional Value (Amount per Serving):
- Calories 297
- Fat 15.3 g
- Carbohydrates 5.1 g
- Sugar 1.4 g
- Protein 33.2 g
- Cholesterol 107 mg

12

LEMON PEPPER CHICKEN BREAST

Preparation Time: 10 minutes
Cooking Time: 30 minutes
Serve: 4

Ingredients:
- 4 chicken breasts, skinless & boneless
- 1 ½ tsp granulated garlic
- 1 tbsp lemon pepper seasoning
- 1 tsp salt

Directions:
1. Preheat the air fryer to 360 F.
2. Rub chicken breasts with garlic and lemon pepper seasoning. Season with salt.
3. Place chicken in the air fryer basket and cook for 30 minutes. Flip chicken halfway through.
4. Serve and enjoy.

Nutritional Value (Amount per Serving):
- Calories 285
- Fat 10.9 g
- Carbohydrates 1.8 g

- Sugar 0.3 g
- Protein 42.6 g
- Cholesterol 130 mg

13

FLAVORFUL CHICKEN FAJITA

Preparation Time: 10 minutes
Cooking Time: 18 minutes
Serve: 4

Ingredients:
- 1 lb chicken breasts, skinless, boneless & sliced
- 1/8 tsp cayenne
- ½ tsp pepper
- 1 tsp cumin
- 2 tsp chili powder
- 2 tsp olive oil
- 1 onion, sliced
- 2 bell pepper, sliced
- 1 tsp salt

Directions:
1. Add chicken and remaining ingredients into the mixing bowl and toss well.
2. Pour chicken mixture into the air fryer basket and cook at 360 F for 16-18 minutes.
3. Stir chicken mixture halfway through.
4. Serve and enjoy.

Nutritional Value (Amount per Serving):
- Calories 272
- Fat 11.3 g
- Carbohydrates 8.2 g
- Sugar 4.3 g
- Protein 34 g
- Cholesterol 101 mg

14

JUICY & CRISPY CHICKEN WINGS

Preparation Time: 10 minutes
Cooking Time: 20 minutes
Serve: 4

Ingredients:
- 1 lb chicken wings
- For rub:
- $1/2$ tsp paprika
- $1/2$ tsp parsley
- $1/2$ tsp dried oregano
- $1/4$ tsp pepper
- 1 tsp smoked paprika
- $1/2$ tsp onion powder
- 1 tsp garlic powder

Directions:

1. Add chicken wings and all rub ingredients into the zip-lock bag, seal bag, and shake well.
2. Add chicken wings into the air fryer basket and cook at 400 F for 20 minutes. Flip chicken wings halfway through.
3. Serve and enjoy.

Nutritional Value (Amount per Serving):

- Calories 222
- Fat 8.5 g
- Carbohydrates 1.4 g
- Sugar 0.4 g
- Protein 33.1 g
- Cholesterol 101 mg

15

SPICE HERB CHICKEN BREAST

Preparation Time: 10 minutes
Cooking Time: 30 minutes
Serve: 2

Ingredients:
- 2 chicken breasts, skinless & boneless
- ¼ tsp red pepper flakes
- ¼ tsp onion powder
- ¼ tsp garlic salt
- ¼ tsp oregano
- ¼ tsp pepper
- 1 tbsp olive oil

Directions:
1. Brush chicken breasts with olive oil.
2. In a small bowl, mix red pepper flakes, onion powder, garlic salt, oregano, and pepper and rub all over chicken breasts.
3. Place chicken breasts into the air fryer basket and cook for 375 F for 25 minutes.
4. Turn chicken breasts and cook for 5 minutes more or until the internal temperature of chicken is reaches to 165 F.
5. Serve and enjoy.

Nutritional Value (Amount per Serving):
- Calories 342
- Fat 17.9 g
- Carbohydrates 0.9 g
- Sugar 0.2 g
- Protein 42.4 g
- Cholesterol 130 mg

16

SPICY MEATBALLS

Preparation Time: 10 minutes
Cooking Time: 12 minutes
Serve: 4

Ingredients:
- 1 lb ground chicken
- 1 egg, lightly beaten
- ½ tsp onion powder
- ¾ tsp garlic powder
- ½ cup hot sauce
- ½ cup breadcrumbs
- ½ tsp salt

Directions:

1. In a mixing bowl, mix chicken, egg, onion powder, garlic powder, ¼ cup hot sauce, breadcrumbs, and salt.

2. Make balls from chicken mixture and place into the air fryer basket and cook at 400 F for 12 minutes.

3. Transfer chicken meatballs into the bowl. Pour remaining hot sauce over meatballs and toss well.

4. Serve and enjoy.

Nutritional Value (Amount per Serving):

- Calories 290
- Fat 10.3 g
- Carbohydrates 10.9 g
- Sugar 1.5 g
- Protein 36.3 g
- Cholesterol 142 mg

17

HERB GARLIC BUTTER CHICKEN WINGS

Preparation Time: 10 minutes
Cooking Time: 20 minutes
Serve: 4

Ingredients:
- 1 lb chicken wings
- For garlic butter:
- 2 tbsp fresh parsley, minced
- ½ tsp garlic powder
- ¼ tsp pepper
- ¼ tsp paprika
- ½ tsp garlic, minced
- ¼ cup butter
- Salt

Directions:
1. Season chicken wings with pepper and salt.
2. Add chicken wings into the air fryer basket and cook at 400 F for 20 minutes. Toss halfway through.
3. Meanwhile, melt butter in a pan over medium heat.
4. Add garlic to the melted butter and sauté for 1 minute. Remove pan from heat.

5. Add parsley, garlic powder, pepper, paprika, and salt into the melted butter.

6. Add chicken wings and melted butter mixture into the large mixing bowl and toss well.

7. Serve and enjoy.

Nutritional Value (Amount per Serving):
- Calories 320
- Fat 20 g
- Carbohydrates 0.7 g
- Sugar 0.1 g
- Protein 33.1 g
- Cholesterol 131 mg

18

FLAVORFUL CHICKEN DRUMSTICKS

Preparation Time: 10 minutes
Cooking Time: 25 minutes
Serve: 4

Ingredients:
- 4 chicken drumsticks
- ½ tsp pepper
- 1 tsp chili powder
- 2 tsp smoked paprika
- 1 tbsp olive oil
- 1 tsp salt

Directions:
1. Add chicken drumsticks into the large mixing bowl.
2. Pour remaining ingredients over chicken drumsticks and toss well.
3. Add chicken drumsticks into the air fryer basket and cook for 390 F for 25 minutes. Turn chicken drumstick halfway through.
4. Serve and enjoy.

Nutritional Value (Amount per Serving):
- Calories 94

- Fat 5.7 g
- Carbohydrates 1.1 g
- Sugar 0.2 g
- Protein 9.8 g
- Cholesterol 30 mg

19

TASTY CHICKEN THIGHS

Preparation Time: 10 minutes
Cooking Time: 28 minutes
Serve: 4
Ingredients:
- 4 chicken thighs
- 2 tbsp hot sauce
- 2 tbsp Cajun seasoning
- 1 tbsp olive oil

Directions:
1. Brush chicken thighs with oil and rub with Cajun seasoning.
2. Place chicken thighs into the air fryer basket and cook at 380 F for 25 minutes.
3. Brush chicken thighs with hot sauce and cook for 3 minutes more.
4. Serve and enjoy.

Nutritional Value (Amount per Serving):
- Calories 271
- Fat 20.5 g
- Carbohydrates 0.1 g

- Sugar 0.1 g
- Protein 20.1 g
- Cholesterol 95 mg

20

ORANGE HONEY CHICKEN WINGS

Preparation Time: 10 minutes
Cooking Time: 20 minutes
Serve: 4

Ingredients:
- 1 lb chicken wings
- For sauce:
- ½ tsp fresh ginger, grated
- 2 tbsp honey
- 2 tbsp soy sauce
- 1 cup orange juice
- Pepper
- Salt

Directions:
1. Season chicken wings with pepper and salt.
2. Add chicken wings into the air fryer basket and cook at 400 F for 20 minutes. Toss halfway through.
3. Meanwhile, add all sauce ingredients into the small saucepan and cook over medium heat until sauce thicken.
4. Add cooked chicken wings into the mixing bowl. Pour sauce over chicken wings and toss well.

5. Serve and enjoy.
Nutritional Value (Amount per Serving):
- Calories 281
- Fat 8.5 g
- Carbohydrates 15.9 g
- Sugar 14 g
- Protein 33.8 g
- Cholesterol 101 mg

21

GARLIC BUTTER TURKEY BREAST

Preparation Time: 10 minutes
Cooking Time: 40 minutes
Serve: 6

Ingredients:
- 2 lbs turkey breast
- 1 tsp rosemary, chopped
- 1 tsp thyme, chopped
- 3 garlic cloves, minced
- 4 tbsp olive oil
- Pepper
- Salt

Directions:
1. Season turkey breast with pepper and salt.
2. In a small bowl, mix oil, rosemary, thyme, and garlic.
3. Brush turkey breast with oil mixture and place into the air fryer basket and cook at 375 F for 40 minutes.
4. Slice and serve.

Nutritional Value (Amount per Serving):
- Calories 229

- Fat 10.2 g
- Carbohydrates 7.1 g
- Sugar 5.3 g
- Protein 26 g
- Cholesterol 85 mg

22

MEATBALLS

Preparation Time: 10 minutes
Cooking Time: 9 minutes
Serve: 4

Ingredients:
- 1 lb ground turkey
- ½ tsp dried oregano
- ½ tsp garlic powder
- 2 tbsp fresh parsley, chopped
- ½ cup breadcrumbs
- 1 egg, lightly beaten
- ¼ cup tomato sauce
- ½ tsp pepper
- ½ tsp salt

Directions:
1. Add all ingredients into the mixing bowl and mix until well combined.
2. Make balls from meat mixture and place into the air fryer basket and cook at 400 F for 9 minutes.
3. Serve and enjoy.

Nutritional Value (Amount per Serving):

- Calories 297
- Fat 14.3 g
- Carbohydrates 11 g
- Sugar 1.7 g
- Protein 34 g
- Cholesterol 157 mg

23

DRY RUB CHICKEN DRUMSTICKS

Preparation Time: 10 minutes
Cooking Time: 20 minutes
Serve: 4
Ingredients:
- 8 chicken drumsticks
- 1 tbsp olive oil
- 1/2 tsp cumin powder
- 1/2 tsp oregano
- 1 tsp garlic powder
- 1/2 tsp onion powder
- 1/2 tsp cayenne pepper
- 1 tsp smoked paprika
- 1 tbsp paprika

Directions:
1. Add chicken drumstick and remaining ingredients into the zip-lock bag, seal bag shake well and place in the refrigerator for 15 minutes.
2. Add chicken drumsticks into the air fryer basket and cook at 400 F for 20 minutes. Flip chicken drumsticks halfway through.
3. Serve and enjoy.

Nutritional Value (Amount per Serving):
- Calories 198
- Fat 9.2 g
- Carbohydrates 2.4 g
- Sugar 0.6 g
- Protein 25.9 g
- Cholesterol 81 mg

24

JUICY LEMON CHICKEN THIGHS

Preparation Time: 10 minutes
Cooking Time: 20 minutes
Serve: 6

Ingredients:
- 6 chicken thighs
- 1 fresh lemon, sliced
- 1 tsp pepper
- 1 tbsp Italian seasoning
- 2 tbsp fresh lemon juice
- 2 tbsp olive oil
- 1 tsp sea salt

Directions:

1. Add chicken thighs, pepper, Italian seasoning, lemon juice, oil, and salt into the zip-lock bag. Seal bag and shake well and place in the refrigerator for 1 hour.

2. Place marinated chicken thighs with lemon slices into the air fryer basket and cook at 350 F for 10 minutes.

3. Flip chicken and cook for 10 minutes more or until the internal temperature of chicken reaches to 165 F.

4. Serve and enjoy.

Nutritional Value (Amount per Serving):
- Calories 289
- Fat 22.4 g
- Carbohydrates 0.6 g
- Sugar 0.3 g
- Protein 20.1 g
- Cholesterol 97 mg

25

EASY & SUPER MOIST CHICKEN WINGS

Preparation Time: 10 minutes
Cooking Time: 20 minutes
Serve: 4

Ingredients:
- 12 chicken wings
- ½ tbsp baking powder
- 1 tsp granulated garlic
- 1 tbsp chili powder
- ½ tsp kosher salt

Directions:
1. Add chicken wings into the large bowl and toss with baking powder, garlic, chili powder, and salt.
2. Add chicken wings into the air fryer basket and cook at 400 F for 20 minutes. Turn chicken wings halfway through.
3. Serve and enjoy.

Nutritional Value (Amount per Serving):
- Calories 486
- Fat 32.4 g
- Carbohydrates 18.5 g

PAMELA KENDRICK

- Sugar 0.3 g
- Protein 29.6 g
- Cholesterol 116 mg

26

ROSEMARY TURKEY BREAST

Preparation Time: 10 minutes
Cooking Time: 50 minutes
Serve: 6

Ingredients:
- 3 lbs turkey breast
- ½ tbsp rosemary
- 1 tbsp olive oil

Directions:
1. Brush turkey breast with oil and place into the air fryer basket and cook at 350 F for 20 minutes.
2. Coat turkey breast with rosemary and cook for 30 minutes more or until the internal temperature of turkey breast reaches to 165 F.
3. Slice and serve.

Nutritional Value (Amount per Serving):
- Calories 257
- Fat 6 g
- Carbohydrates 9 g
- Sugar 8 g

- Protein 38 g
- Cholesterol 98 mg

27

TENDER TURKEY LEGS

Preparation Time: 10 minutes
Cooking Time: 27 minutes
Serve: 4
Ingredients:
- 4 turkey legs
- ¼ tsp oregano
- ¼ tsp rosemary
- 1 tbsp olive oil
- ¼ tsp thyme
- Pepper
- Salt

Directions:
1. In a small bowl, mix oil, thyme, oregano, rosemary, pepper, and salt and rub over turkey legs.
2. Preheat the air fryer to 350 F.
3. Place turkey legs into the air fryer basket and cook for 27 minutes or until internal temperature of turkey legs reaches to 165 F.
4. Serve and enjoy.

Nutritional Value (Amount per Serving):

- Calories 186
- Fat 10 g
- Carbohydrates 0.2 g
- Sugar 0 g
- Protein 22 g
- Cholesterol 88 mg

28

MEATBALLS

Preparation Time: 10 minutes
Cooking Time: 10 minutes
Serve: 4

Ingredients:
- 1 lb ground turkey
- 1 tbsp soy sauce
- ¼ cup fresh parsley
- 1 egg, lightly beaten
- ½ cup breadcrumbs
- Pepper
- Salt

Directions:
1. Add all ingredients into the mixing bowl and mix until well combined.
2. Make balls from meat mixture and place into the air fryer basket and cook at 400 F for 5 minutes.
3. Turn meatballs and cook for 5 minutes more. Cook meatballs in batches.
4. Serve and enjoy.

Nutritional Value (Amount per Serving):

- Calories 294
- Fat 14 g
- Carbohydrates 10 g
- Sugar 1 g
- Protein 34 g
- Cholesterol 157 mg

29

DELICIOUS CHICKEN PATTIES

Preparation Time: 10 minutes
Cooking Time: 12 minutes
Serve: 8

Ingredients:
- 1 lb ground chicken
- ½ tsp Italian seasoning
- ½ tsp garlic powder
- 1 tsp onion powder
- 1 tbsp parsley, chopped
- ½ cup parmesan cheese, grated
- ¼ cup yogurt
- ½ tsp salt

Directions:
1. Add all ingredients into the mixing bowl and mix until well combined.
2. Make equal shapes of patties from meat mixture and place into the air fryer basket.
3. Cook patties at 400 F for 12 minutes. Flip patties halfway through.
4. Serve and enjoy.

Nutritional Value (Amount per Serving):
- Calories 191
- Fat 8 g
- Carbohydrates 1 g
- Sugar 0.7 g
- Protein 22 g
- Cholesterol 66 mg

30

HERB TURKEY BREAST

Preparation Time: 10 minutes
Cooking Time: 40 minutes
Serve: 6

Ingredients:
- 3 lbs turkey breast
- 1 tbsp olive oil
- ¼ tsp herb de Provence
- ½ tsp pepper
- ½ tsp garlic salt

Directions:
1. In a small bowl, mix oil, herb de Provence, pepper, and garlic salt.
2. Brush turkey breast with oil mixture and place into the air fryer basket.
3. Cook turkey breast at 350 F for 40 minutes or until the internal temperature of the turkey reaches to 165 F.
4. Slice and serve.

Nutritional Value (Amount per Serving):
- Calories 257

- Fat 6.1 g
- Carbohydrates 9.8 g
- Sugar 8 g
- Protein 38.8 g
- Cholesterol 98 mg

31

BBQ CHICKEN BREAST

Preparation Time: 10 minutes
Cooking Time: 14 minutes
Serve: 4

Ingredients:
- 4 chicken breasts, skinless & boneless
- 2 tbsp BBQ seasoning

Directions:
1. Rub chicken breasts with BBQ seasoning and let it marinate for 40 minutes.
2. Place chicken breast into the air fryer basket and cook at 400 F for 14 minutes. Flip chicken breasts halfway through.
3. Serve and enjoy.

Nutritional Value (Amount per Serving):
- Calories 277
- Fat 10.8 g
- Carbohydrates 0 g
- Sugar 0 g
- Protein 42.2 g
- Cholesterol 130 mg

32

CHICKEN FRITTERS

Preparation Time: 10 minutes
Cooking Time: 10 minutes
Serve: 4

Ingredients:
- 1 lb ground chicken
- 1/2 tbsp dill, chopped
- 1/2 tsp onion powder
- 1/2 tsp garlic powder
- 1/2 cup parmesan cheese, shredded
- 1/2 cup breadcrumbs
- 2 tbsp green onions, chopped
- Pepper
- Salt

Directions:
1. Add all ingredients into the large bowl and mix until well combined.
2. Make patties from mixture and place into the air fryer basket and cook at 350 F for 10 minutes.
3. Serve and enjoy.

Nutritional Value (Amount per Serving):

- Calories 273
- Fat 9 g
- Carbohydrates 10 g
- Sugar 1 g
- Protein 34 g
- Cholesterol 101 mg

33

GREEK CHICKEN

Preparation Time: 10 minutes
Cooking Time: 35 minutes
Serve: 4

Ingredients:
- 4 lbs whole chicken, cut into pieces
- 2 tsp ground sumac
- 4 garlic cloves, minced
- 2 lemons, sliced
- 2 tbsp olive oil
- 1 tsp lemon zest
- 2 tsp kosher salt

Directions:
1. Brush chicken with oil and rub with sumac, lemon zest, and salt. Marinate in the refrigerator for 3 hours.
2. Add lemon slices into the air fryer basket then add marinated chicken on top.
3. Cook chicken at 350 F for 35 minutes.
4. Serve and enjoy.

Nutritional Value (Amount per Serving):
- Calories 927

- Fat 40 g
- Carbohydrates 1 g
- Sugar 0.1 g
- Protein 131 g
- Cholesterol 404 mg

34

EASY LEMON CHICKEN

Preparation Time: 10 minutes
Cooking Time: 20 minutes
Serve: 4

Ingredients:
- 4 chicken breasts, skinless and boneless
- 1 preserved lemon
- 1 tbsp olive oil

Directions:
1. Add all ingredients into the bowl and mix well. Set aside for 10 minutes.
2. Place chicken into the air fryer basket and cook at 400 F for 20 minutes.
3. Serve and enjoy.

Nutritional Value (Amount per Serving):
- Calories 307
- Fat 14 g
- Carbohydrates 0 g
- Sugar 0 g
- Protein 42 g
- Cholesterol 130 mg

35

MEATBALLS

Preparation Time: 10 minutes
Cooking Time: 10 minutes
Serve: 4

Ingredients:
- 1 lb ground turkey
- ½ cup mushrooms, diced
- 1 tsp fresh thyme, minced
- 1 egg, lightly beaten
- ½ bell pepper, chopped
- Pepper
- Salt

Directions:

1. Add all ingredients into the mixing bowl and mix until well combined.
2. Make balls from meat mixture and place into the air fryer basket and cook at 400 F for 5 minutes.
3. Turn meatballs and cook for 5 minutes more. Cook meatballs in batches.
4. Serve and enjoy.

Nutritional Value (Amount per Serving):

- Calories 672
- Fat 53.4 g
- Carbohydrates 8 g
- Sugar 0 g
- Protein 36 g
- Cholesterol 183 mg

36

GARLIC HERB CHICKEN BREAST

Preparation Time: 10 minutes
Cooking Time: 15 minutes
Serve: 5

Ingredients:
- 2 lbs chicken breasts, skinless and boneless
- 3 garlic cloves, minced
- 1/2 cup yogurt
- 1/4 cup mayonnaise
- 2 tsp garlic herb seasoning
- 1 tsp onion powder
- 1/4 tsp salt

Directions:
1. Preheat the air fryer to 380 F.
2. In a small bowl, mix mayonnaise, seasoning, onion powder, garlic, and yogurt.
3. Brush chicken with mayonnaise mixture and season with salt.
4. Place chicken into the air fryer basket and cook for 15 minutes.
5. Serve and enjoy.

Nutritional Value (Amount per Serving):
- Calories 404
- Fat 17 g
- Carbohydrates 4 g
- Sugar 1 g
- Protein 53 g
- Cholesterol 165 mg

37

MEATBALLS

Preparation Time: 10 minutes
Cooking Time: 10 minutes
Serve: 4

Ingredients:
- 1 lb ground chicken
- 1 tbsp soy sauce
- 1 tbsp hoisin sauce
- 1/2 cup fresh cilantro, chopped
- 2 green onions, chopped
- 1/4 cup shredded coconut
- 1 tsp sesame oil
- 1 tsp sriracha
- Pepper
- Salt

Directions:

1. Add all ingredients into the mixing bowl and mix until well combined.
2. Make balls from meat mixture and place into the air fryer basket and cook at 350 F for 10 minutes. Cook in batches.
3. Serve and enjoy.

Nutritional Value (Amount per Serving):
- Calories 258
- Fat 11 g
- Carbohydrates 3 g
- Sugar 1 g
- Protein 33 g
- Cholesterol 101 mg

38

COCONUT TURKEY MEATBALLS

Preparation Time: 10 minutes
Cooking Time: 12 minutes
Serve: 4

Ingredients:
- 1 egg
- 2 tbsp coconut flour
- 1 lb ground turkey
- 1 garlic clove, minced
- 2 green onion, chopped
- 1/4 cup celery, chopped
- 1/4 cup carrots, grated
- Pepper
- Salt

Directions:
1. Add all ingredients into the mixing bowl and mix until well combined.
2. Make balls from meat mixture and place into the air fryer basket and cook at 400 F for 12 minutes. Turn meatballs halfway through.
3. Serve and enjoy.

Nutritional Value (Amount per Serving):
- Calories 244
- Fat 13 g
- Carbohydrates 2 g
- Sugar 0.7 g
- Protein 32 g
- Cholesterol 157 mg

39

CHEESY CHICKEN MEATBALLS

Preparation Time: 10 minutes
Cooking Time: 10 minutes
Serve: 6

Ingredients:
- 2 eggs
- 2 lbs ground chicken
- 1/4 cup fresh parsley, chopped
- 1/2 cup almond flour
- 1/2 cup ricotta cheese
- 1 tsp pepper
- 2 tsp salt

Directions:
1. Add all ingredients into the mixing bowl and mix until well combined.
2. Make balls from meat mixture and place into the air fryer basket and cook at 380 F for 10 minutes. Cook in batches.
3. Serve and enjoy.

Nutritional Value (Amount per Serving):
- Calories 267

- Fat 9 g
- Carbohydrates 3 g
- Sugar 0.5 g
- Protein 44 g
- Cholesterol 155 mg

40

MEATBALLS

Preparation Time: 10 minutes
Cooking Time: 18 minutes
Serve: 6

Ingredients:
- 1 lb ground turkey
- 1 tsp cumin
- 1/3 cup coconut flour
- 2 cups zucchini, grated
- 1 tsp dried oregano
- 1 tbsp garlic, minced
- 1 tbsp dried onion flakes
- 2 eggs, lightly beaten
- 1 tbsp basil, chopped
- 1 tbsp nutritional yeast
- Pepper
- Salt

Directions:
1. Add all ingredients into the mixing bowl and mix until well combined.

2.Make balls from meat mixture and place into the air fryer basket and cook at 400 F for 18 minutes. Cook in batches.

3.Serve and enjoy.

Nutritional Value (Amount per Serving):
- Calories 188
- Fat 10 g
- Carbohydrates 3 g
- Sugar 1 g
- Protein 24 g
- Cholesterol 132 mg

LEAN & GREEN PORK

41

EASY PORK PATTIES

Preparation Time: 10 minutes
Cooking Time: 35 minutes
Serve: 6

Ingredients:
- 2 lbs ground pork
- 1 egg, lightly beaten
- 1 onion, minced
- 1 carrot, minced
- 1/2 cup breadcrumbs
- 1 tsp garlic powder
- 1 tsp paprika
- Pepper
- Salt

Directions:
1. Add all ingredients into the large bowl and mix until well combined.
2. Make patties from mixture and place into the air fryer basket and cook at 375 F for 20 minutes.
3. Turn patties and cook for 15 minutes more.
4. Serve and enjoy.

Nutritional Value (Amount per Serving):
- Calories 276
- Fat 6 g
- Carbohydrates 9 g
- Sugar 2 g
- Protein 42 g
- Cholesterol 138 mg

42

LEMON PEPPER PORK CHOPS

Preparation Time: 10 minutes
Cooking Time: 15 minutes
Serve: 4

Ingredients:
- 4 pork chops, boneless
- 1 tsp lemon pepper seasoning
- Salt

Directions:
1. Season pork chops with lemon pepper seasoning and salt.
2. Place pork chops into the air fryer basket and cook at 400 F for 15 minutes.
3. Serve and enjoy.

Nutritional Value (Amount per Serving):
- Calories 257
- Fat 19 g
- Carbohydrates 0.3 g
- Sugar 0 g
- Protein 18 g
- Cholesterol 69 mg

43

MEATBALLS

Preparation Time: 10 minutes
Cooking Time: 20 minutes
Serve: 6

Ingredients:
- 16 oz ground pork
- 1/2 onion, diced
- 1 egg, lightly beaten
- 1/4 cup parmesan cheese, grated
- 1/4 cup parsley, chopped
- 1 tsp garlic, minced
- 1/2 cup breadcrumbs
- Pepper
- Salt

Directions:
1. Add all ingredients into the mixing bowl and mix until well combined.
2. Make balls from meat mixture and place into the air fryer basket and cook at 400 F for 20 minutes. Cook in batches.
3. Serve and enjoy.

Nutritional Value (Amount per Serving):

- Calories 176
- Fat 5 g
- Carbohydrates 7 g
- Sugar 1 g
- Protein 23 g
- Cholesterol 89 mg

44

CRISPY CRUSTED PARMESAN PORK CHOPS

Preparation Time: 10 minutes
Cooking Time: 30 minutes
Serve: 3

Ingredients:
- 2 tbsp milk
- 1 egg, lightly beaten
- 3 pork chops, boneless
- 3 tbsp parmesan cheese, grated
- 1/2 cup crackers, crushed
- Pepper
- Salt

Directions:
1. In a shallow bowl, whisk egg and milk.
2. In a separate dish, mix cheese, crackers, pepper, and salt.
3. Dip pork chops in egg then coat with cheese mixture.
4. Place coated pork chops into the air fryer basket and cook at 350 F for 30 minutes.
5. Serve and enjoy.

Nutritional Value (Amount per Serving):
- Calories 334

- Fat 24 g
- Carbohydrates 6 g
- Sugar 0.8 g
- Protein 20 g
- Cholesterol 124 mg

45

SPICY PORK STEAK

Preparation Time: 10 minutes
Cooking Time: 15 minutes
Serve: 4

Ingredients:
- 1 lb pork steaks, boneless
- 1 tsp garam masala
- 4 garlic cloves
- 1 tbsp ginger, sliced
- 1/2 onion, diced
- 1/2 tsp cayenne
- 1/2 tsp ground cardamom
- 1 tsp cinnamon
- 1 tsp ground fennel
- 1 tsp salt

Directions:
1. Add all ingredients except meat into the blender and blend until smooth.
2. Add the meat into the bowl.
3. Pour blended mixture over the meat and mix well.
4. Place meat into the refrigerator for overnight.

5. Place marinated meat into the air fryer basket and cook at 330 F for 15 minutes. Turn halfway through.

6. Slice and serve.

Nutritional Value (Amount per Serving):
- Calories 313
- Fat 19 g
- Carbohydrates 4 g
- Sugar 0.7 g
- Protein 29 g
- Cholesterol 108 mg

46

DASH PORK CHOPS

Preparation Time: 10 minutes
Cooking Time: 20 minutes
Serve: 2

Ingredients:
- 2 pork chops, boneless
- 1 tbsp dash seasoning

Directions:
1. Rub seasoning all over the pork chops.
2. Place pork chops into the air fryer basket and cook at 360 F for 20 minutes. Turn halfway through.
3. Serve and enjoy.

Nutritional Value (Amount per Serving):
- Calories 256
- Fat 19 g
- Carbohydrates 0 g
- Sugar 0 g
- Protein 18 g
- Cholesterol 69 mg

47

JUICY PORK CHOPS

Preparation Time: 10 minutes
Cooking Time: 13 minutes
Serve: 4

Ingredients:
- 4 pork chops, boneless
- 1/2 tsp granulated onion
- 1/2 tsp granulated garlic
- 1/2 tsp celery seeds
- 1/2 tsp parsley
- 2 tsp olive oil
- 1/2 tsp salt

Directions:

1. In a small bowl, mix seasonings and sprinkle onto the pork chops.
2. Place pork chops into the air fryer basket and cook at 350 F for 5 minutes.
3. Turn pork chops and cook for 8 minutes more.
4. Serve and enjoy.

Nutritional Value (Amount per Serving):
- Calories 278

- Fat 22 g
- Carbohydrates 0.4 g
- Sugar 0.1 g
- Protein 18 g
- Cholesterol 69 mg

48

CREOLE PORK CHOPS

Preparation Time: 10 minutes
Cooking Time: 12 minutes
Serve: 6

Ingredients:
- 1 1/2 lbs pork chops, boneless
- 1/4 cup parmesan cheese, grated
- 1/3 cup almond flour
- 1 tsp paprika
- 1 tsp Creole seasoning
- 1 tsp garlic powder

Directions:
1. Preheat the air fryer to 360 F.
2. Add all ingredients except pork chops into the zip-lock bag.
3. Add pork chops into the bag, seal bag, and shake well.
4. Place pork chops into the air fryer basket and cook for 12 minutes.
5. Serve and enjoy.

Nutritional Value (Amount per Serving):
- Calories 365

- Fat 28 g
- Carbohydrates 0.5 g
- Sugar 0.2 g
- Protein 25 g
- Cholesterol 98 mg

49

CAJUN PORK CHOPS

Preparation Time: 10 minutes
Cooking Time: 9 minutes
Serve: 2

Ingredients:
- 2 pork chops, boneless
- 1 tsp paprika
- 3 tbsp parmesan cheese, grated
- 1/3 cup almond flour
- 1/2 tsp Cajun seasoning
- 1 tsp herb de Provence

Directions:
1. Preheat the air fryer to 350 F.
2. Mix almond flour, Cajun seasoning, herb de Provence, paprika, and parmesan cheese.
3. Coat both the pork chops with almond flour mixture.
4. Place pork chops into the air fryer basket and cook for 9 minutes.
5. Serve and enjoy.

Nutritional Value (Amount per Serving):
- Calories 259

- Fat 20 g
- Carbohydrates 0.6 g
- Sugar 0.1 g
- Protein 18 g
- Cholesterol 69 mg

50

FLAVORFUL LEMON GARLIC PORK CHOPS

Preparation Time: 10 minutes
Cooking Time: 20 minutes
Serve: 5

Ingredients:
- 2 lbs pork chops
- 2 tbsp fresh lemon juice
- 2 tbsp garlic, minced
- 1 tbsp fresh parsley
- 1 1/2 tbsp olive oil
- Pepper
- Salt

Directions:
1. Add pork chops into the zip-lock bag.
2. In a small bowl, mix garlic, parsley, olive oil, lemon juice, pepper, and salt and pour over pork chops into the zip-lock bag.
3. Seal bag and place in the refrigerator for 30 minutes.
4. Add marinated pork chops into the air fryer basket and cook at 400 F for 10 minutes.
5. Turn pork chops and cook for 10 minutes more.
6. Serve and enjoy.

Nutritional Value (Amount per Serving):
- Calories 623
- Fat 49 g
- Carbohydrates 1.3 g
- Sugar 0.2 g
- Protein 41 g
- Cholesterol 156 mg

51

THYME GARLIC PORK CHOPS

Preparation Time: 10 minutes
Cooking Time: 15 minutes
Serve: 8

Ingredients:
- 8 pork chops, boneless
- 1 tsp thyme
- 2 tbsp olive oil
- 1/4 tsp pepper
- 1 tbsp parsley
- 6 garlic cloves, minced
- 3/4 cup parmesan cheese
- 1/2 tsp sea salt

Directions:
1. Preheat the air fryer to 400 F.
2. In a bowl, mix oil, spices, and parmesan cheese.
3. Brush oil mixture over pork chops.
4. Place pork chops into the air fryer basket and cook for 10 minutes.
5. Turn pork chops and cook for 10 minutes more.
6. Serve and enjoy.

Nutritional Value (Amount per Serving):
- Calories 315
- Fat 26 g
- Carbohydrates 0.9 g
- Sugar 0 g
- Protein 18 g
- Cholesterol 76 mg

52

PESTO PORK CHOPS

Preparation Time: 10 minutes
Cooking Time: 18 minutes
Serve: 5

Ingredients:
- 5 pork chops
- 1 tbsp basil pesto
- 2 tbsp almond flour

Directions:
1. Brush pork chops with pesto and sprinkle with almond flour.
2. Place pork chops into the air fryer basket and cook at 350 F for 18 minutes.
3. Serve and enjoy.

Nutritional Value (Amount per Serving):
- Calories 256
- Fat 19 g
- Carbohydrates 0 g
- Sugar 0 g
- Protein 18 g
- Cholesterol 69 mg

53

SPICY GARLIC PORK CHOPS

Preparation Time: 10 minutes
Cooking Time: 14 minutes
Serve: 2

Ingredients:
- 2 pork chops
- 1/2 tbsp garlic, minced
- 1/2 tsp sesame oil
- 1/4 cup hot sauce
- Pepper
- Salt

Directions:
1. Preheat the air fryer to 350 F.
2. Add all ingredients into the bowl and mix well and place in the refrigerator for 1 hour.
3. Place pork chops into the air fryer basket and cook for 14 minutes. Turn halfway through.
4. Serve and enjoy.

Nutritional Value (Amount per Serving):
- Calories 269

- Fat 21 g
- Carbohydrates 0.7 g
- Sugar 0 g
- Protein 18 g
- Cholesterol 69 mg

54

MEATBALLS

Preparation Time: 10 minutes
Cooking Time: 15 minutes
Serve: 4

Ingredients:
- 4 oz sausage meat
- 1/2 tsp garlic paste
- 1/2 onion, diced
- 3 tbsp almond flour
- 1 tsp sage
- Pepper
- Salt

Directions:
1. Preheat the air fryer to 350 F.
2. Add all ingredients into the mixing bowl and mix until well combined.
3. Make balls from meat mixture and place into the air fryer basket and cook for 15 minutes. Cook in batches.
4. Serve and enjoy.

Nutritional Value (Amount per Serving):
- Calories 91

Lean & Green Pork

- Fat 7 g
- Carbohydrates 1.5 g
- Sugar 0.6 g
- Protein 5 g
- Cholesterol 21 mg

55

FLAVORFUL SPICY PORK CHOPS

Preparation Time: 10 minutes
Cooking Time: 10 minutes
Serve: 4

Ingredients:
- 4 pork chops
- 1 1/2 tsp olive oil
- 1/2 tsp ground cumin
- 1 tsp paprika
- 1/2 tsp dried sage
- 1/2 tsp cayenne pepper
- 1/2 tsp black pepper
- 1/2 tsp garlic salt

Directions:
1. Preheat the air fryer to 400 F.
2. In a small bowl, mix paprika, garlic salt, sage, pepper, cayenne pepper, and cumin.
3. Rub pork chops with spice mixture and place into the air fryer basket.
4. Cook pork chops for 10 minutes. Turn halfway through.
5. Serve and enjoy.

Nutritional Value (Amount per Serving):
- Calories 276
- Fat 21 g
- Carbohydrates 1 g
- Sugar 0.2 g
- Protein 18 g
- Cholesterol 69 mg

LEAN & GREEN SEAFOOD

56

FLAVORFUL PRAWNS

Preparation Time: 10 minutes
Cooking Time: 6 minutes
Serve: 4

Ingredients:
- 12 king prawns
- 1/2 tsp black pepper
- 1 tsp chili powder
- 1 tsp red chili flakes
- 1 tbsp vinegar
- 1 tbsp ketchup
- 3 tbsp mayonnaise
- 1/2 tsp sea salt

Directions:
1. Preheat the air fryer to 350 F.
2. Add prawns, chili flakes, chili powder, black pepper, and salt to the bowl and toss well.
3. Add shrimp to the air fryer basket and cook for 6 minutes.
4. In a small bowl, mix mayo, ketchup, and vinegar.
5. Serve shrimp with mayo mixture and enjoy.

Nutritional Value (Amount per Serving):

- Calories 275
- Fat 5 g
- Carbohydrates 6.5 g
- Sugar 1.6 g
- Protein 47.1 g
- Cholesterol 3 mg

57

LEMON GARLIC SHRIMP

Preparation Time: 10 minutes
Cooking Time: 5 minutes
Serve: 4

Ingredients:
- 1 lb shrimp, peeled
- 1 tbsp olive oil
- 1 lemon juice
- 1 lemon zest
- 1/4 cup fresh parsley, chopped
- 4 garlic cloves, minced
- 1/4 tsp red pepper flakes
- 1/4 tsp sea salt

Directions:
1. Preheat the air fryer to 400 F.
2. Add all ingredients except parsley and lemon juice into the bowl and toss well.
3. Add shrimp mixture to the air fryer basket and cook for 5 minutes. Shake halfway through.
4. Add parsley and lemon juice. Toss well.
5. Serve and enjoy.

Nutritional Value (Amount per Serving):
- Calories 171
- Fat 5 g
- Carbohydrates 3 g
- Sugar 0.1 g
- Protein 26 g
- Cholesterol 239 mg

58

OLD BAY SPICY SHRIMP

Preparation Time: 10 minutes
Cooking Time: 6 minutes
Serve: 2

Ingredients:
- 1/2 lb shrimp, peeled and deveined
- 1/2 tsp old bay seasoning
- 1 tbsp olive oil
- 1/4 tsp paprika
- 1 tsp cayenne pepper
- 1/8 tsp salt

Directions:
1. Preheat the air fryer to 390 F.
2. Add all ingredients into the bowl and toss well.
3. Add shrimp mixture into the air fryer basket and cook for 6 minutes.
4. Serve and enjoy.

Nutritional Value (Amount per Serving):
- Calories 198
- Fat 9.1 g

- Carbohydrates 2.3 g
- Sugar 0.1 g
- Protein 26 g
- Cholesterol 239 mg

59

LEMON GARLIC SALMON

Preparation Time: 10 minutes
Cooking Time: 11 minutes
Serve: 2

Ingredients:
- 2 salmon fillets
- 1/4 cup white wine
- 2 tsp garlic, minced
- 2 tbsp olive oil
- 2 tbsp fresh lemon juice
- Pepper
- Salt

Directions:
1. Preheat the air fryer to 350 F.
2. Season salmon with pepper and salt and place into the air fryer basket and cook for 6 minutes.
3. Meanwhile, in a saucepan, add remaining ingredients and heat over low heat for 5 minutes.
4. Transfer salmon on serving dish then pour prepared sauce over salmon.
5. Serve and enjoy.

Nutritional Value (Amount per Serving):
- Calories 380
- Fat 23 g
- Carbohydrates 2 g
- Sugar 0.6 g
- Protein 35 g
- Cholesterol 109 mg

60

PARMESAN HERB CRUST SALMON

Preparation Time: 10 minutes
Cooking Time: 10 minutes
Serve: 5

Ingredients:
- 5 salmon fillets
- 1/4 cup fresh parsley, chopped
- 3 garlic cloves, minced
- 3/4 cup parmesan cheese, shredded
- 1 tsp BBQ seasoning
- 1 tsp paprika
- 1 tbsp olive oil
- Pepper
- Salt

Directions:
1. Preheat the air fryer to 425 F.
2. Add salmon, seasoning, and olive oil to the bowl and mix well.
3. Place salmon fillet into the air fryer basket.
4. In a bowl, mix cheese, garlic, and parsley.

5. Sprinkle cheese mixture on top of salmon and cook for 10 minutes.

6. Serve and enjoy.

Nutritional Value (Amount per Serving):
- Calories 264
- Fat 13 g
- Carbohydrates 1 g
- Sugar 0.1 g
- Protein 34.8 g
- Cholesterol 78 mg

61

SIMPLE PAPRIKA SALMON

Preparation Time: 10 minutes
Cooking Time: 15 minutes
Serve: 4

Ingredients:
- 4 salmon fillets
- 1/4 tsp garlic powder
- 1/2 tsp smoked paprika
- 1/4 tsp salt

Directions:
1. In a small bowl, mix together paprika, garlic, and salt.
2. Rub paprika mixture on top of salmon.
3. Place salmon fillet into the air fryer basket and cook at 350 F for 15 minutes.
4. Serve and enjoy.

Nutritional Value (Amount per Serving):
- Calories 237
- Fat 11 g
- Carbohydrates 0.3 g
- Sugar 0.1 g

- Protein 34.6 g
- Cholesterol 78 mg

62

CRAB PATTIES

Preparation Time: 10 minutes
Cooking Time: 10 minutes
Serve: 4

Ingredients:
- 1 egg
- 12 oz crabmeat
- 2 green onion, chopped
- 1/4 cup mayonnaise
- 1 cup almond flour
- 1 tsp old bay seasoning
- 1 tsp red pepper flakes
- 1 tbsp fresh lemon juice

Directions:
1. Preheat the air fryer to 400 F.
2. Add half almond flour into the mixing bowl. Add remaining ingredients and mix until well combined.
3. Make patties from mixture and coat with remaining almond flour and place into the air fryer basket.
4. Cook patties for 5 minutes. Turn patties cook for 5 minutes more.

5. Serve and enjoy.

Nutritional Value (Amount per Serving):
- Calories 159
- Fat 6.5 g
- Carbohydrates 17 g
- Sugar 6.6 g
- Protein 8.2 g
- Cholesterol 62 mg

63

AIR FRIED CATFISH FILLETS

Preparation Time: 10 minutes
Cooking Time: 20 minutes
Serve: 4

Ingredients:
- 4 catfish fillets
- 1 tbsp olive oil
- 4 tbsp fish seasoning
- 1 tbsp fresh parsley, chopped

Directions:
1. Preheat the air fryer to 400 F.
2. Brush fish fillets with oil and season with fish seasoning.
3. Place fish fillets into the air fryer basket and cook for 10 minutes.
4. Flip fish fillets and cook for 10 minutes more.
5. Garnish with parsley and serve.

Nutritional Value (Amount per Serving):
- Calories 246
- Fat 15 g
- Carbohydrates 0.1 g

PAMELA KENDRICK

- Sugar 0 g
- Protein 24 g
- Cholesterol 75 mg

64

SIMPLE LIME GARLIC SHRIMP

Preparation Time: 10 minutes
Cooking Time: 8 minutes
Serve: 2

Ingredients:
- 1 cup shrimp
- 1 garlic clove, minced
- 1 fresh lime juice
- Pepper
- Salt

Directions:
1. Preheat the air fryer to 350 F.
2. Add all ingredients into the bowl and toss well.
3. Add shrimp mixture into the air fryer basket and cook for 8 minutes. stir halfway through.
4. Serve and enjoy.

Nutritional Value (Amount per Serving):
- Calories 59
- Fat 0.6 g
- Carbohydrates 0.5 g

- Sugar 0 g
- Protein 12 g
- Cholesterol 111 mg

65

CRISPY COCONUT SHRIMP

Preparation Time: 10 minutes
Cooking Time: 5 minutes
Serve: 4

Ingredients:
- 2 egg whites
- 15 oz shrimp, peeled
- 1/4 tsp cayenne pepper
- 1/2 cup shredded coconut
- 1/2 cup almond flour
- 1/2 tsp salt

Directions:
1. Preheat the air fryer to 400 F.
2. Whisk egg whites in a shallow dish.
3. In a bowl, mix shredded coconut, almond flour, and cayenne pepper.
4. Dip shrimp into the egg mixture then coat with coconut mixture and place into the air fryer basket and cook for 5 minutes.
5. Serve and enjoy.

Nutritional Value (Amount per Serving):
- Calories 179

- Fat 5 g
- Carbohydrates 3.4 g
- Sugar 0.8 g
- Protein 28 g
- Cholesterol 239 mg

66

BASIL PARMESAN SHRIMP

Preparation Time: 10 minutes
Cooking Time: 10 minutes
Serve: 6

Ingredients:
- 2 lbs shrimp, peeled and deveined
- 2/3 cup parmesan cheese, grated
- 3 garlic cloves, minced
- 2 tbsp olive oil
- 1 tsp onion powder
- 1 tsp basil
- 1/2 tsp oregano
- 1 tsp pepper

Directions:
1. Add all ingredients into the large bowl and toss well.
2. Add shrimp mixture into the air fryer basket and cook at 350 F for 10 minutes.
3. Serve and enjoy.

Nutritional Value (Amount per Serving):
- Calories 225

- Fat 7.3 g
- Carbohydrates 3.4 g
- Sugar 0.2 g
- Protein 34.6 g
- Cholesterol 318 mg

67

PARMESAN CAJUN SHRIMP

Preparation Time: 10 minutes
Cooking Time: 5 minutes
Serve: 4

Ingredients:
- 1 lb shrimp
- 1 tsp olive oil
- 1 tbsp Cajun seasoning
- 2 tbsp parmesan cheese
- 2 garlic cloves, minced
- 1/2 cup almond flour

Directions:
1. Add all ingredients into the large bowl and toss well.
2. Transfer shrimp to the air fryer basket and cook at 390 F for 5 minutes. Shake basket 2 times.
3. Serve and enjoy.

Nutritional Value (Amount per Serving):
- Calories 147
- Fat 3.1 g
- Carbohydrates 2.2 g

- Sugar 0 g
- Protein 26 g
- Cholesterol 239 mg

68

SRIRACHA SHRIMP

Preparation Time: 10 minutes
Cooking Time: 8 minutes
Serve: 4

Ingredients:
- 1 lb shrimp, peeled
- 1 tbsp ketchup
- 3 tbsp mayonnaise
- 1/2 tsp paprika
- 1 tsp sriracha
- 1 tbsp garlic, minced
- 1/2 tsp salt

Directions:
1. In a bowl, mix mayonnaise, paprika, sriracha, garlic, ketchup, and salt.
2. Add shrimp to the bowl and stir well.
3. Add shrimp into the air fryer basket and cook at 325 F for 8 minutes. Shake halfway through.
4. Serve and enjoy.

Nutritional Value (Amount per Serving):
- Calories 187

- Fat 5 g
- Carbohydrates 6.4 g
- Sugar 1.6 g
- Protein 26 g
- Cholesterol 242 mg

69

CHILI GARLIC SHRIMP

Preparation Time: 10 minutes
Cooking Time: 7 minutes
Serve: 4

Ingredients:
- 1 lb shrimp, peeled and deveined
- 1 red chili, sliced
- 1 lemon, sliced
- 1/2 tsp garlic powder
- 1 tbsp olive oil
- Pepper
- Salt

Directions:
1. Preheat the air fryer to 400 F.
2. Add all ingredients into the bowl and toss well.
3. Transfer shrimp mixture into the air fryer basket and cook for 5 minutes.
4. Shake basket and cook for 2 minutes more.
5. Serve and enjoy.

Nutritional Value (Amount per Serving):
- Calories 166

- Fat 5.4 g
- Carbohydrates 2 g
- Sugar 0.1 g
- Protein 25 g
- Cholesterol 239 mg

70

QUICK SALMON PATTIES

Preparation Time: 10 minutes
Cooking Time: 10 minutes
Serve: 2

Ingredients:
- 1 egg
- 14 oz salmon
- 1/2 cup almond flour
- 1/4 cup onion, diced
- 1 tsp dill weed
- Pepper
- Salt

Directions:
1. Add all ingredients into the mixing bowl and mix well.
2. Make patties from bowl mixture and place into the air fryer basket and cook at 370 F for 5 minutes.
3. Turn patties and cook for 5 minutes more.
4. Serve and enjoy.

Nutritional Value (Amount per Serving):
- Calories 310

- Fat 14 g
- Carbohydrates 1.8 g
- Sugar 0.8 g
- Protein 42.9 g
- Cholesterol 172 mg

71

DELICIOUS ASIAN SHRIMP

Preparation Time: 10 minutes
Cooking Time: 10 minutes
Serve: 4

Ingredients:
- 1 lb shrimp, peeled and deveined
- 2 garlic cloves, minced
- 2 tbsp soy sauce
- 2 tbsp Thai chili sauce
- 1 tbsp arrowroot
- 1 tsp sesame seeds
- 1 tbsp green onion, sliced
- 1/8 tsp ginger, minced

Directions:

1. Toss shrimp with arrowroot and transfer into the air fryer basket.
2. Cook shrimp for 5 minutes. Shake basket and cook shrimp for 5 minutes more.
3. Meanwhile, in a bowl, mix soy sauce, ginger, garlic, and chili sauce.
4. Add shrimp to the bowl and mix well.

5. Garnish with green onions and sesame seeds.
6. Serve and enjoy.

Nutritional Value (Amount per Serving):
- Calories 147
- Fat 2.3 g
- Carbohydrates 3.4 g
- Sugar 0.2 g
- Protein 26.7 g
- Cholesterol 239 mg

72

GARLIC ROSEMARY SHRIMP

Preparation Time: 10 minutes
Cooking Time: 10 minutes
Serve: 4

Ingredients:
- 1 lb shrimp, peeled and deveined
- 1 garlic clove, minced
- 1/2 tbsp fresh rosemary, chopped
- 1 tbsp olive oil
- Pepper
- Salt

Directions:
1. Add shrimp and remaining ingredients in a bowl and toss well.
2. Add shrimp mixture into the air fryer basket and cook at 400 F for 10 minutes.
3. Serve and enjoy.

Nutritional Value (Amount per Serving):
- Calories 167
- Fat 5.5 g

- Carbohydrates 2.3 g
- Sugar 0 g
- Protein 25 g
- Cholesterol 239 mg

73

GREEK SHRIMP

Preparation Time: 10 minutes
Cooking Time: 25 minutes
Serve: 4

Ingredients:
- 1 lb shrimp, peeled
- 1 tbsp garlic, sliced
- 2 cups grape tomatoes
- 1 tbsp olive oil
- Pepper
- Salt

Directions:
1. Add shrimp, oil, garlic, tomatoes, pepper, and salt into the bowl and toss well.
2. Transfer shrimp mixture into the air fryer basket and cook at 400 F for 25 minutes.
3. Serve and enjoy.

Nutritional Value (Amount per Serving):
- Calories 184
- Fat 5 g

- Carbohydrates 5.9 g
- Sugar 2.4 g
- Protein 26.8 g
- Cholesterol 239 mg

74

SIMPLE CAJUN SHRIMP

Preparation Time: 10 minutes
Cooking Time: 10 minutes
Serve: 4

Ingredients:
- 1 lb shrimp, deveined & peeled
- 3/4 tbsp Cajun seasoning
- 2 tbsp olive oil
- Salt

Directions:
1. Add shrimp, Cajun seasoning, and oil into the mixing bowl and toss well.
2. Add shrimp into the air fryer basket and cook at 325 F for 10 minutes.
3. Serve and enjoy.

Nutritional Value (Amount per Serving):
- Calories 195
- Fat 8 g
- Carbohydrates 1.7 g
- Sugar 0 g

- Protein 25 g
- Cholesterol 239 mg

75

SPICY LEMON SHRIMP

Preparation Time: 10 minutes
Cooking Time: 6 minutes
Serve: 4

Ingredients:
- 1 lb shrimp
- 1 tsp lemon zest, grated
- 1 tsp steak seasoning
- 1/4 tsp red pepper flakes
- 2 garlic cloves, minced
- 1 tbsp parsley, chopped
- 2 tsp fresh lemon juice
- 2 tsp olive oil
- Pepper
- Salt

Directions:

1. Add shrimp and remaining ingredients into the bowl and toss well.

2. Add shrimp into the air fryer basket and cook at 400 F for 6 minutes.

3. Serve and enjoy.

Nutritional Value (Amount per Serving):
- Calories 159
- Fat 4 g
- Carbohydrates 2.5 g
- Sugar 0.1 g
- Protein 26 g
- Cholesterol 239 mg

76

LEMON PEPPER TILAPIA

Preparation Time: 10 minutes
Cooking Time: 10 minutes
Serve: 2
Ingredients:
- 2 tilapia fillets
- 1/2 tsp lemon pepper seasoning
- 1/2 tsp garlic powder
- 1/2 tsp onion powder
- Salt

Directions:
1. Season fish fillets with garlic powder, onion powder, lemon pepper seasoning, and salt.
2. Place fish fillets in the air fryer basket and cook at 360 F for 10 minutes.
3. Serve and enjoy.

Nutritional Value (Amount per Serving):
- Calories 76
- Fat 1 g
- Carbohydrates 1.3 g

- Sugar 0.4 g
- Protein 16.2 g
- Cholesterol 43 mg

77

HERB TUNA PATTIES

Preparation Time: 10 minutes
Cooking Time: 10 minutes
Serve: 10

Ingredients:
- 2 eggs, lightly beaten
- 14.5 oz can tuna, drained and flaked
- 1/2 tsp dried herbs
- 3 tbsp parmesan cheese, grated
- 1/2 cup breadcrumbs
- 1 tbsp lemon juice
- 1/2 tsp garlic powder
- 2 tbsp onion, minced
- 1 celery stalk, chopped
- Pepper
- Salt

Directions:
1. Add all ingredients into the mixing bowl and mix until well combined.
2. Make patties from tuna mixture and place into the air fryer

basket and cook at 360 F for 10 minutes. Turn patties halfway through.

3.Serve and enjoy.

Nutritional Value (Amount per Serving):
- Calories 85
- Fat 1.5 g
- Carbohydrates 4.4 g
- Sugar 0.6 g
- Protein 12 g
- Cholesterol 46 mg

78

SIMPLE CAJUN SALMON

Preparation Time: 10 minutes
Cooking Time: 8 minutes
Serve: 4

Ingredients:
- 4 salmon fillets
- 1 tsp Cajun seasoning
- 4 tbsp olive oil

Directions:
1. Brush salmon fillets with oil and season with Cajun seasoning.
2. Place salmon fillets into the air fryer basket and cook at 375 F for 8 minutes.
3. Serve and enjoy.

Nutritional Value (Amount per Serving):
- Calories 337
- Fat 22 g
- Carbohydrates 0 g
- Sugar 0 g
- Protein 34 g
- Cholesterol 109 mg

79

QUICK SALMON BURGER PATTIES

Preparation Time: 10 minutes
Cooking Time: 7 minutes
Serve: 2

Ingredients:
- 8 oz salmon fillet, minced
- 1/4 tsp garlic powder
- 1 egg, lightly beaten
- 1/4 tsp onion powder
- 1/4 tsp paprika
- Pepper
- Salt

Directions:
1. Add all ingredients into the bowl and mix until well combined.
2. Make patties from mixture and place into the air fryer basket and cook at 390 F for 7 minutes.
3. Serve and enjoy.

Nutritional Value (Amount per Serving):
- Calories 183

- Fat 9 g
- Carbohydrates 0.5 g
- Sugar 0.3 g
- Protein 24 g
- Cholesterol 132 mg

80

HERB FISH FILLETS

Preparation Time: 10 minutes
Cooking Time: 5 minutes
Serve: 2

Ingredients:
- 2 salmon fillets
- 2 tbsp olive oil
- 1/4 tsp smoked paprika
- 1 tsp herb de Provence
- Pepper
- Salt

Directions:

1. Brush salmon fillets with oil and sprinkle with paprika, herb de Provence, pepper, and salt.
2. Place salmon fillets in the air fryer basket and cook at 390 F for 5 minutes.
3. Serve and enjoy.

Nutritional Value (Amount per Serving):
- Calories 407
- Fat 30 g

- Carbohydrates 0.2 g
- Sugar 0 g
- Protein 34 g
- Cholesterol 94 mg

81

MARINATED ASIAN SALMON

Preparation Time: 10 minutes
Cooking Time: 10 minutes
Serve: 2

Ingredients:
- 2 salmon fillets, skinless and boneless
- For marinade:
- 2 tbsp scallions, minced
- 2 tbsp mirin
- 2 tbsp soy sauce
- 1 tbsp olive oil
- 1 tbsp ginger, grated
- 2 garlic cloves, minced

Directions:
1. Add all marinade ingredients into the zip-lock bag and mix well.
2. Add salmon in a zip-lock bag.
3. Seal bag and shake well and places it in the refrigerator for 1 hour.
4. Place marinated salmon fillets into the air fryer basket and cook at 360 F for 10 minutes.

5. Serve and enjoy.

Nutritional Value (Amount per Serving):
- Calories 345
- Fat 18.2 g
- Carbohydrates 11.6 g
- Sugar 4.5 g
- Protein 36.1 g
- Cholesterol 78 mg

82

OLD BAY SALMON

Preparation Time: 10 minutes
Cooking Time: 8 minutes
Serve: 4

Ingredients:
- 4 salmon fillets
- 1 tsp old bay seasoning
- 1/4 cup olive oil
- Pepper
- Salt

Directions:
1. Brush salmon fillets with oil and season with old bay seasoning, pepper, and salt.
2. Place salmon fillets in the air fryer basket and cook at 375 F for 8 minutes.
3. Serve and enjoy.

Nutritional Value (Amount per Serving):
- Calories 337
- Fat 22.5 g
- Carbohydrates 0 g

- Sugar 0 g
- Protein 34.7 g
- Cholesterol 109 mg

83

LEMON PEPPER WHITE FISH

Preparation Time: 10 minutes
Cooking Time: 10 minutes
Serve: 2

Ingredients:
- 2 white fish fillets
- 1 tbsp olive oil
- 1/2 tsp lemon pepper seasoning
- 1/2 tsp garlic powder
- 1/4 tsp smoked paprika
- 1/2 tsp onion powder
- Salt

Directions:
1. Brush fish fillets with oil and season with paprika, garlic powder, onion powder, lemon pepper seasoning, and salt.
2. Place fish fillets into the air fryer basket and cook at 360 F for 10 minutes.
3. Serve and enjoy.

Nutritional Value (Amount per Serving):
- Calories 100

- Fat 1.1 g
- Carbohydrates 1.3 g
- Sugar 0.4 g
- Protein 21.3 g
- Cholesterol 55 mg

84

DELICIOUS HERB SALMON

Preparation Time: 10 minutes
Cooking Time: 15 minutes
Serve: 4

Ingredients:
- 1 lb salmon fillets
- 1/4 tsp dried basil
- 1 tbsp dried chives
- 1/4 tsp dried thyme
- 1/2 tbsp dried rosemary
- 1 tbsp olive oil
- Pepper
- Salt

Directions:
1. In a small bowl, mix olive oil, thyme, basil, chives, and rosemary.
2. Brush salmon with oil mixture.
3. Place salmon in the air fryer basket and cook at 400 F for 15 minutes.
4. Serve and enjoy.

Nutritional Value (Amount per Serving):

Lean & Green Seafood

- Calories 182
- Fat 10.6 g
- Carbohydrates 0.4 g
- Sugar 0 g
- Protein 22.1 g
- Cholesterol 50 mg

85

FLAVORFUL SPICY SHRIMP

Preparation Time: 10 minutes

Cooking Time: 6 minutes

Serve: 4

Ingredients:
- 1 lb shrimp, peeled and deveined
- 1/4 tsp chili powder
- 2 tsp smoked paprika
- 1/4 tsp cayenne
- 2 tbsp olive oil
- 1 tsp dried oregano
- 1 tsp garlic powder
- 1 tsp onion powder
- Pepper
- Salt

Directions:

1. In a bowl, toss shrimp with remaining ingredients.

2. Add shrimp into the air fryer basket and cook at 400 F for 6 minutes.

3. Serve and enjoy.

Nutritional Value (Amount per Serving):

- Calories 205
- Fat 9.2 g
- Carbohydrates 3.7 g
- Sugar 0.5 g
- Protein 26.2 g
- Cholesterol 239 mg

86

SIMPLE SHRIMP FAJITAS

Preparation Time: 10 minutes
Cooking Time: 20 minutes
Serve: 10

Ingredients:
- 1 lb shrimp
- 2 bell peppers, diced
- 2 tbsp taco seasoning
- 1/2 cup onion, diced
- 1 tbsp olive oil

Directions:

1. Add shrimp and remaining ingredients into the bowl and toss well.

2. Add shrimp mixture into the air fryer basket and cook at 390 F for 20 minutes.

3. Serve and enjoy.

Nutritional Value (Amount per Serving):
- Calories 75
- Fat 2.2 g
- Carbohydrates 3 g

- Sugar 1.4 g
- Protein 10.6 g
- Cholesterol 96 mg

87

LEMON PEPPER BASA

Preparation Time: 10 minutes
Cooking Time: 12 minutes
Serve: 4

Ingredients:
- 4 basa fish fillets
- 1/2 tsp garlic powder
- 1/4 tsp lemon pepper seasoning
- 4 tbsp fresh lemon juice
- 8 tsp olive oil
- Pepper
- Salt

Directions:
1. Brush fish fillets with oil and season with garlic powder, lemon pepper seasoning, pepper, and salt.
2. Place fish fillets in the air fryer basket and cook at 400 F for 12 minutes.
3. Drizzle lemon juice over cooked fish fillets and serve.

Nutritional Value (Amount per Serving):
- Calories 308

- Fat 21.4 g
- Carbohydrates 5.5 g
- Sugar 3.4 g
- Protein 24.1 g
- Cholesterol 0 mg

88

SPICY HALIBUT

Preparation Time: 10 minutes
Cooking Time: 12 minutes
Serve: 4

Ingredients:
- 1 lb halibut fillets
- 1/2 tsp smoked paprika
- 1/4 tsp garlic powder
- 1/4 cup olive oil
- 1/4 tsp chili powder
- Pepper
- Salt

Directions:
1. In a small bowl, mix together oil, chili powder, garlic powder, paprika, pepper, and salt.
2. Brush fish fillets with oil mixture.
3. Place fish fillets in the air fryer basket and cook at 400 F for 12 minutes.
4. Serve and enjoy.

Nutritional Value (Amount per Serving):
- Calories 235

- Fat 15.3 g
- Carbohydrates 0.3 g
- Sugar 0.1 g
- Protein 23.9 g
- Cholesterol 36 mg

89

AIR FRY CATFISH FILLETS

Preparation Time: 10 minutes
Cooking Time: 15 minutes
Serve: 4

Ingredients:
- 1 lb catfish fillets, cut 1/2-inch thick
- 1 tbsp dried oregano, crushed
- 1/2 tsp ground cumin
- 1/2 tsp chili powder
- 1 tsp crushed red pepper
- 2 tsp onion powder
- Pepper
- Salt

Directions:
1. In a small bowl, mix cumin, chili powder, crushed red pepper, onion powder, oregano, pepper, and salt.
2. Rub fish fillets with the spice mixture and place in air fryer basket and cook at 350 F for 20 minutes.
3. Serve and enjoy.

Nutritional Value (Amount per Serving):
- Calories 165

Lean & Green Seafood

- Fat 8.9 g
- Carbohydrates 2.3 g
- Sugar 0.6 g
- Protein 18 g
- Cholesterol 53 mg

90

LEMON GARLIC SWORDFISH

Preparation Time: 10 minutes

Cooking Time: 10 minutes

Serve: 2

Ingredients:
- 12 oz swordfish fillets
- 3 tbsp olive oil
- 1/2 tsp lemon zest, grated
- 1/2 tsp ginger, grated
- 1/8 tsp crushed red pepper
- 1 garlic clove, minced
- 2 tsp fresh parsley, chopped

Directions:

1. In a small bowl, mix 2 tbsp oil, lemon zest, red pepper, ginger, garlic, and parsley.
2. Season fish fillets with salt.
3. Heat remaining oil in a pan over medium-high heat.
4. Place fish fillets in the pan and cook until browned.
5. Transfer fish fillets to the air fryer basket and cook at 400 F for 10 minutes.
6. Pour oil mixture over fish fillets and serve.

Nutritional Value (Amount per Serving):
- Calories 450
- Fat 29.8 g
- Carbohydrates 1.1 g
- Sugar 0.1 g
- Protein 43.4 g
- Cholesterol 85 mg

91

SIMPLE GARLIC TILAPIA

Preparation Time: 10 minutes

Cooking Time: 15 minutes

Serve: 4

Ingredients:
- 1 lb tilapia fillets
- 2 tbsp dried parsley
- 2 tbsp garlic, minced
- 2 tbsp olive oil
- Pepper
- Salt

Directions:

1. In a small bowl, mix oil, garlic, pepper, and salt.
2. Brush fish fillets with oil mixture and place into the air fryer basket and cook at 375 F for 15 minutes.
3. Garnish with parsley and serve.

Nutritional Value (Amount per Serving):
- Calories 160
- Fat 8.1 g
- Carbohydrates 1.5 g

- Sugar 0.1 g
- Protein 21.4 g
- Cholesterol 55 mg

92

SPICY COD

Preparation Time: 10 minutes
Cooking Time: 10 minutes
Serve: 2

Ingredients:
- 1 lb cod fillets
- 1 tbsp fresh parsley, chopped
- 1 1/2 tbsp olive oil
- 1 tbsp fresh lemon juice
- 1/8 tsp cayenne pepper
- 1/4 tsp chili powder
- 1/4 tsp salt

Directions:

1. Brush fish fillets with oil and lemon juice and season with cayenne pepper, chili powder, and salt.

2. Place fish fillets into the air fryer basket and cook at 375 F for 10 minutes.

3. Garnish with parsley and serve.

Nutritional Value (Amount per Serving):
- Calories 275

- Fat 12.7 g
- Carbohydrates 0.5 g
- Sugar 0.2 g
- Protein 40.7 g
- Cholesterol 111 mg

93

GARLIC ROSEMARY SHRIMP

Preparation Time: 10 minutes
Cooking Time: 10 minutes
Serve: 4

Ingredients:
- 1 lb shrimp, peeled and deveined
- 1/2 tbsp fresh rosemary, chopped
- 1 tbsp olive oil
- 2 garlic cloves, minced
- Pepper
- Salt

Directions:

1. Add shrimp and remaining ingredients in a large bowl and toss well.
2. Pour shrimp mixture into the air fryer basket and cook at 375 F for 10 minutes.
3. Serve and enjoy.

Nutritional Value (Amount per Serving):
- Calories 165
- Fat 5.5 g

- Carbohydrates 2.5 g
- Sugar 0 g
- Protein 26 g
- Cholesterol 239 mg

94

FLAVORS PARMESAN SHRIMP

Preparation Time: 10 minutes
Cooking Time: 10 minutes
Serve: 4

Ingredients:
- 1 lb shrimp, peeled and deveined
- 1 tbsp olive oil
- 1/4 tsp oregano
- 1/2 tsp pepper
- 1/4 cup parmesan cheese, grated
- 4 garlic cloves, minced
- 1/2 tsp onion powder
- 1/2 tsp basil

Directions:
1. Add all ingredients into the large bowl and toss well.
2. Add shrimp to the air fryer basket and cook at 350 F for 10 minutes.
3. Serve and enjoy.

Nutritional Value (Amount per Serving):
- Calories 190

- Fat 6.7 g
- Carbohydrates 3.4 g
- Sugar 0.1 g
- Protein 27.9 g
- Cholesterol 243 mg

95

SHRIMP WITH VEGETABLES

Preparation Time: 10 minutes
Cooking Time: 15 minutes
Serve: 4

Ingredients:
- 1 lb shrimp, peeled and deveined
- 1 bell pepper, sliced
- 1 zucchini, sliced
- 1/4 cup parmesan cheese, grated
- 1 tbsp Italian seasoning
- 1 tbsp garlic, minced
- 1 tbsp olive oil
- Pepper
- Salt

Directions:
1. Add all ingredients into the bowl and toss well.
2. Transfer shrimp mixture into the air fryer basket and cook at 390 F for 15 minutes.
3. Serve and enjoy.

Nutritional Value (Amount per Serving):
- Calories 215

- Fat 7.9 g
- Carbohydrates 6.9 g
- Sugar 2.7 g
- Protein 28.7 g
- Cholesterol 245 mg

GREEN & SIDE DISHES

96

HEALTHY & TASTY GREEN BEANS

Preparation Time: 10 minutes
Cooking Time: 10 minutes
Serve: 2

Ingredients:
- 2 cups green beans
- 1/8 tsp ground allspice
- 1/4 tsp ground cinnamon
- 1/2 tsp dried oregano
- 2 tbsp olive oil
- 1/4 tsp ground coriander
- 1/4 tsp ground cumin
- 1/8 tsp cayenne pepper
- 1/2 tsp salt

Directions:
1. Add all ingredients into the bowl and toss well.
2. Add green beans into the air fryer basket and cook at 370 F for 10 minutes. Shake basket halfway through
3. Serve and enjoy.

Nutritional Value (Amount per Serving):
- Calories 158

- Fat 14 g
- Carbohydrates 8.6 g
- Sugar 1.6 g
- Protein 2.1 g
- Cholesterol 0 mg

97

CHEESY BRUSSELS SPROUTS

Preparation Time: 10 minutes
Cooking Time: 12 minutes
Serve: 4

Ingredients:
- 1 lb Brussels sprouts, cut stems and halved
- 1/4 cup parmesan cheese, grated
- 1 tbsp olive oil
- 1/4 tsp garlic powder
- Pepper
- Salt

Directions:
1. Preheat the air fryer to 350 F.
2. Toss Brussels sprouts, oil, garlic powder, pepper, and salt into the bowl.
3. Transfer Brussels sprouts into the air fryer basket and cook for 12 minutes.
4. Top with cheese and serve.

Nutritional Value (Amount per Serving):
- Calories 132

- Fat 7 g
- Carbohydrates 10 g
- Sugar 2.5 g
- Protein 7 g
- Cholesterol 8 mg

98

GARLIC CAULIFLOWER FLORETS

Preparation Time: 10 minutes
Cooking Time: 20 minutes
Serve: 4

Ingredients:
- 4 cups cauliflower florets
- 1/2 tsp cumin powder
- 1/2 tsp coriander powder
- 5 garlic cloves, chopped
- 4 tablespoons olive oil
- 1/2 tsp salt

Directions:
1. Add all ingredients into the bowl and toss well.
2. Add cauliflower florets into the air fryer basket and cook at 400 F for 20 minutes. Shake halfway through.
3. Serve and enjoy.

Nutritional Value (Amount per Serving):
- Calories 153
- Fat 14 g
- Carbohydrates 7 g

PAMELA KENDRICK

- Sugar 2.5 g
- Protein 2.3 g
- Cholesterol 0 mg

99

DELICIOUS RATATOUILLE

Preparation Time: 10 minutes

Cooking Time: 15 minutes

Serve: 6

Ingredients:
- 1 eggplant, diced
- 3 garlic cloves, chopped
- 1 onion, diced
- 3 tomatoes, diced
- 2 bell peppers, diced
- 1 tbsp vinegar
- 1 1/2 tbsp olive oil
- 2 tbsp herb de Provence
- Pepper
- Salt

Directions:
1. Preheat the air fryer to 400 F.
2. Add all ingredients into the bowl and toss well.
3. Add vegetable mixture into the air fryer basket and cook for 15 minutes. Stir halfway through.
4. Serve and enjoy.

Nutritional Value (Amount per Serving):
- Calories 83
- Fat 4 g
- Carbohydrates 12 g
- Sugar 6 g
- Protein 2 g
- Cholesterol 0 mg

100

SIMPLE GREEN BEANS

Preparation Time: 10 minutes
Cooking Time: 10 minutes
Serve: 4

Ingredients:
- 2 cups green beans
- 1 tsp olive oil
- Pepper
- Salt

Directions:
1. In a bowl, toss green beans with oil. Season with pepper and salt.
2. Transfer green beans into the air fryer basket and cook at 390 F for 10 minutes.
3. Serve and enjoy.

Nutritional Value (Amount per Serving):
- Calories 27
- Fat 1.2 g
- Carbohydrates 3.9 g
- Sugar 0.8 g

PAMELA KENDRICK

- Protein 1 g
- Cholesterol 0 mg

101

AIR FRYER TOFU

Preparation Time: 10 minutes

Cooking Time: 15 minutes

Serve: 4

Ingredients:

- 15 oz extra firm tofu, cut into bite-sized pieces
- 1 tbsp olive oil
- 2 tbsp soy sauce
- 1 garlic clove, minced
- Pepper
- Salt

Directions:

1. Add tofu, garlic, oil, soy sauce, pepper, and salt in a bowl and toss well. Set aside for 15 minutes.

2. Add tofu pieces into the air fryer basket and cook at 370 F for 15 minutes.

3. Serve and enjoy.

Nutritional Value (Amount per Serving):

- Calories 115
- Fat 8 g

- Carbohydrates 2 g
- Sugar 0.8 g
- Protein 9.8 g
- Cholesterol 0 mg

102

HEALTHY ZUCCHINI PATTIES

Preparation Time: 10 minutes
Cooking Time: 30 minutes
Serve: 6

Ingredients:
- 1 cup zucchini, shredded and squeeze out all liquid
- 1 egg, lightly beaten
- 1/4 tsp red pepper flakes
- 1/4 cup parmesan cheese, grated
- 1/2 tbsp Dijon mustard
- 1/2 tbsp mayonnaise
- 1/2 cup breadcrumbs
- 2 tbsp onion, minced
- Pepper
- Salt

Directions:
1. Add all ingredients into the bowl and mix until well combined.
2. Make patties from mixture and place into the basket and cook at 375 F for 15 minutes.
3. Turn patties and cook for 15 minutes more.

4.Serve and enjoy.
Nutritional Value (Amount per Serving):
- Calories 80
- Fat 3 g
- Carbohydrates 8 g
- Sugar 1 g
- Protein 4 g
- Cholesterol 33 mg

103

HEALTHY ASPARAGUS SPEARS

Preparation Time: 10 minutes
Cooking Time: 15 minutes
Serve: 4

Ingredients:
- 35 asparagus spears, cut the ends
- 1/2 tsp garlic powder
- 1 tbsp olive oil
- 1/4 tsp onion powder
- Pepper
- Salt

Directions:
1. Add asparagus into the large bowl. Drizzle with oil.
2. Sprinkle with onion powder, garlic powder, pepper, and salt. Toss well.
3. Arrange asparagus into the air fryer basket and cook at 375 F for 15 minutes.
4. Serve and enjoy.

Nutritional Value (Amount per Serving):
- Calories 75

- Fat 4 g
- Carbohydrates 8 g
- Sugar 4 g
- Protein 4 g
- Cholesterol 0 mg

104

SPICY BRUSSELS SPROUTS

Preparation Time: 10 minutes
Cooking Time: 14 minutes
Serve: 2

Ingredients:
- 1/2 lb Brussels sprouts, trimmed and halved
- 1/2 tsp chili powder
- 1/4 tsp cayenne
- 1/2 tbsp olive oil
- 1/4 tsp smoked paprika
- Pepper
- Salt

Directions:
1. Add all ingredients into the large bowl and toss well.
2. Add Brussels sprouts into the air fryer basket and cook at 370 F for 14 minutes.
3. Serve and enjoy.

Nutritional Value (Amount per Serving):
- Calories 82
- Fat 4 g

- Carbohydrates 10 g
- Sugar 2 g
- Protein 4 g
- Cholesterol 0 mg

105

CHEESE BROCCOLI FRITTERS

Preparation Time: 10 minutes
Cooking Time: 30 minutes
Serve: 4
Ingredients:
- 2 eggs, lightly beaten
- 3 cups broccoli florets, cook & mashed
- 2 cups cheddar cheese
- 1/4 cup almond flour
- 2 garlic cloves, minced
- Pepper
- Salt

Directions:
1. Add all ingredients into the bowl and mix until combined.
2. Make patties from mixture and place into the basket and cook at 350 F for 15 minutes.
3. Turn patties and cook for 15 minutes more.
4. Serve and enjoy.

Nutritional Value (Amount per Serving):
- Calories 285

- Fat 21 g
- Carbohydrates 6 g
- Sugar 1.6 g
- Protein 18 g
- Cholesterol 141 mg

106

AIR FRYER BELL PEPPERS

Preparation Time: 10 minutes
Cooking Time: 8 minutes
Serve: 3

Ingredients:
- 3 cups bell peppers, cut into pieces
- 1 tsp olive oil
- 1/4 tsp onion powder
- 1/4 tsp garlic powder
- Pepper
- Salt

Directions:
1. Add all ingredients into the large bowl and toss well.
2. Transfer bell peppers into the air fryer basket and cook at 360 F for 8 minutes. Stir halfway through.
3. Serve and enjoy.

Nutritional Value (Amount per Serving):
- Calories 52
- Fat 2 g
- Carbohydrates 9 g

- Sugar 6 g
- Protein 1.2 g
- Cholesterol 0 mg

107

AIR FRIED TASTY EGGPLANT

Preparation Time: 10 minutes
Cooking Time: 12 minutes
Serve: 2

Ingredients:
- 1 eggplant, cut into cubes
- 1/4 tsp oregano
- 1 tbsp olive oil
- 1/2 tsp garlic powder
- 1/4 tsp chili powder

Directions:
1. Add all ingredients into the large bowl and toss well.
2. Transfer eggplant into the air fryer basket and cook at 390 F for 12 minutes. Stir halfway through.
3. Serve and enjoy.

Nutritional Value (Amount per Serving):
- Calories 120
- Fat 7 g
- Carbohydrates 14 g
- Sugar 7 g

- Protein 2 g
- Cholesterol 0 mg

108

ASIAN GREEN BEANS

Preparation Time: 10 minutes
Cooking Time: 10 minutes
Serve: 2
Ingredients:
- 8 oz green beans, trimmed and cut in half
- 1 tbsp tamari
- 1 tsp sesame oil

Directions:
1. Add all ingredients into the large bowl and toss well.
2. Add green beans into the air fryer basket and cook at 400 F for 10 minutes.
3. Serve and enjoy.

Nutritional Value (Amount per Serving):
- Calories 60
- Fat 2 g
- Carbohydrates 8 g
- Sugar 1 g
- Protein 3 g
- Cholesterol 0 mg

109

SPICY ASIAN BRUSSELS SPROUTS

Preparation Time: 10 minutes
Cooking Time: 15 minutes
Serve: 4

Ingredients:
- 1 lb Brussels sprouts, cut in half
- 1 tbsp gochujang
- 1 1/2 tbsp olive oil
- 1/2 tsp salt

Directions:
1. In a bowl, mix olive oil, gochujang, and salt.
2. Add Brussels sprouts into the bowl and toss until well coated.
3. Add Brussels sprouts into the air fryer basket and cook at 360 F for 15 minutes.
4. Serve and enjoy.

Nutritional Value (Amount per Serving):
- Calories 94
- Fat 5 g
- Carbohydrates 10 g
- Sugar 2 g

- Protein 4 g
- Cholesterol 0 mg

110

HEALTHY MUSHROOMS

Preparation Time: 10 minutes
Cooking Time: 12 minutes
Serve: 2

Ingredients:
- 8 oz mushrooms, clean and cut into quarters
- 1 tbsp fresh parsley, chopped
- 1 tsp soy sauce
- 1/2 tsp garlic powder
- 1/4 tsp onion powder
- 1 tbsp olive oil
- Pepper
- Salt

Directions:
1. Add mushrooms and remaining ingredients into the bowl and toss well.
2. Add mushrooms into the air fryer basket and cook at 380 F for 12 minutes. Stir halfway through.
3. Serve and enjoy.

Nutritional Value (Amount per Serving):
- Calories 90

- Fat 7 g
- Carbohydrates 4 g
- Sugar 2 g
- Protein 4 g
- Cholesterol 0 mg

111

CHEESE STUFF PEPPERS

Preparation Time: 10 minutes
Cooking Time: 8 minutes
Serve: 4

Ingredients:
- 10 jalapeno peppers, halved, remove seeds and stem
- 1/2 cup cheddar cheese, shredded
- 1/2 cup Monterey jack cheese, shredded
- 8 oz cream cheese, softened

Directions:
1. In a bowl, mix together Monterey jack cheese and cream cheese.
2. Stuff cheese mixture into jalapeno halved.
3. Place jalapeno pepper into the air fryer basket and cook at 370 F for 8 minutes.
4. Serve and enjoy.

Nutritional Value (Amount per Serving):
- Calories 365
- Fat 33.1 g
- Carbohydrates 5.4 g

- Sugar 1.4 g
- Protein 13.2 g
- Cholesterol 90 mg

112

CHEESY BROCCOLI CAULIFLOWER

Preparation Time: 10 minutes
Cooking Time: 20 minutes
Serve: 6

Ingredients:
- 4 cups cauliflower florets
- 4 cups broccoli florets
- 2/3 cup parmesan cheese, shredded
- 5 garlic cloves, minced
- 1/3 cup olive oil
- Pepper
- Salt

Directions:
1. Add half cheese, broccoli, cauliflower, garlic, oil, pepper, and salt into the bowl and toss well.
2. Add broccoli and cauliflower to air fryer basket and cook at 370 F for 20 minutes.
3. Add remaining cheese. Toss well.
4. Serve and enjoy.

Nutritional Value (Amount per Serving):
- Calories 165

- Fat 13.6 g
- Carbohydrates 8.6 g
- Sugar 2.7 g
- Protein 6.4 g
- Cholesterol 7 mg

113

AIR FRYER BROCCOLI & BRUSSELS SPROUTS

Preparation Time: 10 minutes
Cooking Time: 30 minutes
Serve: 6

Ingredients:
- 1 lb Brussels sprouts, cut ends
- 1 lb broccoli, cut into florets
- 1/2 onion, chopped
- 1 tsp paprika
- 1 tsp garlic powder
- 1/2 tsp pepper
- 3 tbsp olive oil
- 3/4 tsp salt

Directions:
1. Add all ingredients into the bowl and toss well.
2. Add vegetable mixture into the air fryer basket and cook at 370 F for 30 minutes.
3. Serve and enjoy.

Nutritional Value (Amount per Serving):
- Calories 125

- Fat 7.6 g
- Carbohydrates 13.4 g
- Sugar 3.5 g
- Protein 5 g
- Cholesterol 0 mg

114

SPICY ASPARAGUS SPEARS

Preparation Time: 10 minutes
Cooking Time: 15 minutes
Serve: 4

Ingredients:
- 35 asparagus spears, cut the ends
- 1/2 tsp chili powder
- 1/4 tsp paprika
- 1 tbsp olive oil
- Pepper
- Salt

Directions:
1. Add asparagus into the large bowl. Drizzle with oil.
2. Sprinkle with paprika, chili powder, pepper, and salt. Toss well.
3. Add asparagus into the air fryer basket and cook at 400 F for 15 minutes.
4. Serve and enjoy.

Nutritional Value (Amount per Serving):
- Calories 75

- Fat 3.8 g
- Carbohydrates 8.4 g
- Sugar 4 g
- Protein 4.7 g
- Cholesterol 0 mg

115

STUFFED MUSHROOMS

Preparation Time: 10 minutes
Cooking Time: 8 minutes
Serve: 16

Ingredients:
- 16 mushrooms, clean and chop stems
- 2 garlic cloves, minced
- 1/2 tsp chili powder
- 1/4 tsp onion powder
- 1/4 cup cheddar cheese, shredded
- 2 oz crab meat, chopped
- 8 oz cream cheese, softened
- 1/4 tsp pepper

Directions:

1. In a bowl, mix cheese, mushroom stems, chili powder, onion powder, pepper, crabmeat, cream cheese, and garlic until well combined.

2. Stuff mushrooms with cheese mixture and place into the air fryer basket and cook at 370 F for 8 minutes.

3. Serve and enjoy.

Nutritional Value (Amount per Serving):

- Calories 65
- Fat 5.7 g
- Carbohydrates 1.3 g
- Sugar 0.4 g
- Protein 2.6 g
- Cholesterol 19 mg

116

BROCCOLI TOTS

Preparation Time: 10 minutes
Cooking Time: 15 minutes
Serve: 4

Ingredients:
- 2 cups broccoli florets, cooked & mash
- 1/4 cup almond flour
- 2 egg whites
- 1 cup cheddar cheese, shredded
- 1/8 tsp salt

Directions:
1. Preheat the air fryer to 325 F.
2. Add all ingredients into the bowl mix until well combined.
3. Make small tots from mixture and place into the air fryer basket and cook for 15 minutes.
4. Serve and enjoy.

Nutritional Value (Amount per Serving):
- Calories 148
- Fat 10.4 g
- Carbohydrates 3.9 g

- Sugar 1.1 g
- Protein 10.5 g
- Cholesterol 30 mg

117

CHEESY JALAPENO PEPPER

Preparation Time: 10 minutes
Cooking Time: 5 minutes
Serve: 5

Ingredients:
- 10 fresh jalapeno peppers, cut in half and remove seeds
- 1/4 tsp onion powder
- 1/4 tsp garlic powder
- 1/4 tsp chili powder
- 1/4 cup mozzarella cheese, shredded
- 6 oz cream cheese, softened

Directions:

1. In a bowl, mix cream cheese, chili powder, garlic powder, onion powder, and mozzarella cheese.
2. Stuff each jalapeno half with a cheese mixture.
3. Place stuffed peppers in the air fryer basket and cook at 370 F for 5 minutes.
4. Serve and enjoy.

Nutritional Value (Amount per Serving):
- Calories 216

- Fat 18.9 g
- Carbohydrates 3.4 g
- Sugar 1.1 g
- Protein 8.6 g
- Cholesterol 56 mg

118

TASTY EGGPLANT SLICES

Preparation Time: 10 minutes
Cooking Time: 20 minutes
Serve: 4

Ingredients:
- 1 eggplant, cut into 1-inch slices
- 1/2 tsp Italian seasoning
- 1 tsp paprika
- 2 tbsp olive oil
- 1/8 tsp cayenne
- 1/2 tsp red pepper
- 1 tsp garlic powder

Directions:
1. Add all ingredients into the large bowl and toss well.
2. Place eggplant slices into the basket and cook at 375 F for 20 minutes. Turn halfway through.
3. Serve and enjoy.

Nutritional Value (Amount per Serving):
- Calories 100
- Fat 7.5 g

- Carbohydrates 8.8 g
- Sugar 4.5 g
- Protein 1.5 g
- Cholesterol 0 mg

119

HEALTHY ZUCCHINI CHIPS

Preparation Time: 10 minutes
Cooking Time: 16 minutes
Serve: 2

Ingredients:
- 1 zucchini, cut into slices
- 1 tbsp olive oil
- 1 tsp Cajun seasoning
- Pepper
- Salt

Directions:
1. Add all ingredients into the bowl and toss well.
2. Add zucchini slices into the air fryer basket and cook at 370 F for 16 minutes. Turn halfway through.
3. Serve and enjoy.

Nutritional Value (Amount per Serving):
- Calories 75
- Fat 7.2 g
- Carbohydrates 3.3 g
- Sugar 1.7 g

- Protein 1.2 g
- Cholesterol 0 mg

120

ROSEMARY BASIL MUSHROOMS

Preparation Time: 10 minutes
Cooking Time: 14 minutes
Serve: 4

Ingredients:
- 1 lb mushroom caps
- 1 garlic clove, minced
- 1/2 tbsp vinegar
- 1/2 tsp ground coriander
- 1 tsp rosemary, chopped
- 1 tbsp basil, minced
- Pepper
- Salt

Directions:
1. Add all ingredients into the bowl and toss well.
2. Add mushrooms into the air fryer basket and cook at 350 F for 14 minutes.
3. Serve and enjoy.

Nutritional Value (Amount per Serving):
- Calories 28

- Fat 0.4 g
- Carbohydrates 4.2 g
- Sugar 2 g
- Protein 3.6 g
- Cholesterol 0 mg

30-DAY MEAL PLAN

Day 1
    Breakfast- Cheesy Egg Bites
    Lunch- Flavorful Prawns
    Dinner- Flavorful Spicy Pork Chops

Day 2
    Breakfast- Egg & Pepper
    Lunch- Delicious No Breading Chicken Breast
    Dinner- Crispy Crusted Parmesan Pork Chops

Day 3
    Breakfast- Spinach Egg Muffins
    Lunch- Lemon Garlic Shrimp
    Dinner- Pesto Pork Chops

Day 4
    Breakfast- Parmesan Spinach Egg Muffins
    Lunch- Lemon Pepper Chicken Breast
    Dinner- Spicy Garlic Pork Chops

Day 5
    Breakfast- Cheddar Kale Egg Cups
    Lunch- Old Bay Spicy Shrimp
    Dinner- Thyme Garlic Pork Chops

Day 6
Breakfast- Mushroom Spinach Egg Muffins
Lunch- Flavorful Chicken Fajita
Dinner- Flavorful Lemon Garlic Pork Chops
Day 7
Breakfast- Easy Scrambled Eggs
Lunch- Air Fried Catfish Fillets
Dinner- Cajun Pork Chops
Day 8
Breakfast- Egg & Tomato
Lunch- Spice Herb Chicken Breast
Dinner- Creole Pork Chops
Day 9
Breakfast- Healthy Spinach Frittata
Lunch- Crab Patties
Dinner- Juicy Pork Chops
Day 10
Breakfast- Vegetable Egg Muffins
Lunch- Herb Turkey Breast
Dinner- Dash Pork Chops
Day 11
Breakfast- Cheesy Egg Bites
Lunch- Simple Paprika Salmon
Dinner- Spicy Pork Steak
Day 12
Breakfast- Egg & Pepper
Lunch- BBQ Chicken Breast
Dinner- Crispy Crusted Parmesan Pork Chops
Day 13
Breakfast- Spinach Egg Muffins
Lunch- Parmesan Herb Crust Salmon
Dinner- Flavorful Spicy Pork Chops
Day 14
Breakfast- Parmesan Spinach Egg Muffins
Lunch- Garlic Herb Chicken Breast
Dinner- Lemon Pepper Pork Chops

Day 15
Breakfast- Cheddar Kale Egg Cups
Lunch- Lemon Garlic Salmon
Dinner- Easy Pork Patties
Day 16
Breakfast- Cheesy Egg Bites
Lunch- Flavorful Prawns
Dinner- Flavorful Spicy Pork Chops
Day 17
Breakfast- Egg & Pepper
Lunch- Delicious No Breading Chicken Breast
Dinner- Crispy Crusted Parmesan Pork Chops
Day 18
Breakfast- Spinach Egg Muffins
Lunch- Lemon Garlic Shrimp
Dinner- Pesto Pork Chops
Day 19
Breakfast- Parmesan Spinach Egg Muffins
Lunch- Lemon Pepper Chicken Breast
Dinner- Spicy Garlic Pork Chops
Day 20
Breakfast- Cheddar Kale Egg Cups
Lunch- Old Bay Spicy Shrimp
Dinner- Thyme Garlic Pork Chops
Day 21
Breakfast- Mushroom Spinach Egg Muffins
Lunch- Flavorful Chicken Fajita
Dinner- Flavorful Lemon Garlic Pork Chops
Day 22
Breakfast- Easy Scrambled Eggs
Lunch- Air Fried Catfish Fillets
Dinner- Cajun Pork Chops
Day 23
Breakfast- Egg & Tomato
Lunch- Spice Herb Chicken Breast
Dinner- Creole Pork Chops

Day 24
Breakfast- Healthy Spinach Frittata
Lunch- Crab Patties
Dinner- Juicy Pork Chops
Day 25
Breakfast- Vegetable Egg Muffins
Lunch- Herb Turkey Breast
Dinner- Dash Pork Chops
Day 26
Breakfast- Cheesy Egg Bites
Lunch- Simple Paprika Salmon
Dinner- Spicy Pork Steak
Day 27
Breakfast- Egg & Pepper
Lunch- BBQ Chicken Breast
Dinner- Crispy Crusted Parmesan Pork Chops
Day 28
Breakfast- Spinach Egg Muffins
Lunch- Parmesan Herb Crust Salmon
Dinner- Flavorful Spicy Pork Chops
Day 29
Breakfast- Parmesan Spinach Egg Muffins
Lunch- Garlic Herb Chicken Breast
Dinner- Lemon Pepper Pork Chops
Day 30
Breakfast- Cheddar Kale Egg Cups
Lunch- Lemon Garlic Salmon
Dinner- Easy Pork Patties

CONCLUSION

The Optavia diet is driven and introduces by Medifast, is a famous food substitute company. The Optavia diet program requires feed you low carb and low-calorie food. The Optavia diet is one of the effective weight loss which reduces your weight rapidly and offers you long term weight loss benefits.

The cookbook contains 120 Optavia recipes written from different categories like breakfast, lean and green poultry, lean and green pork, lean and green seafood, and green & side. All the recipes written in this book are unique and written into easily understandable form with step by step instructions. It also comes with preparation and cooking time. All the recipes end with their nutritional value information.

www.ingramcontent.com/pod-product-compliance
Lightning Source LLC
Chambersburg PA
CBHW071603080526
44588CB00010B/1007